the art of Seduction

Also by Robert Greene
The 48 Laws of Power

the art of 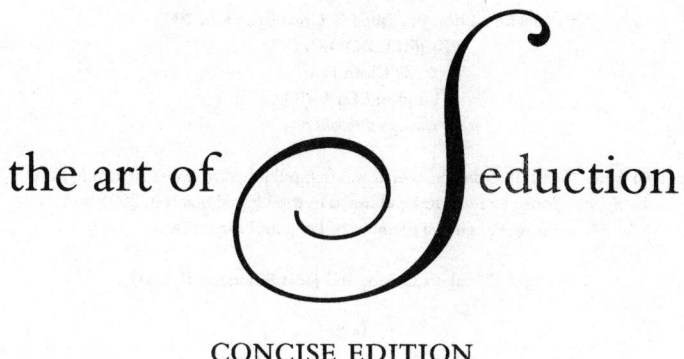 eduction

CONCISE EDITION

Robert Greene

A Joost Elffers Book

P
PROFILE BOOKS

This concise edition published in Great Britain in 2003 by
PROFILE BOOKS LTD
29 Cloth Fair
London EC1A 7JQ
www.profilebooks.com

Derived from *The Art of Seduction*, which was first published in Great Britain in 2001 by Profile Books and was first published in the United States in 2001 by Viking Penguin, a member of Penguin Putnam Inc.

Copyright © Robert Greene and Joost Elffers, 2001, 2003

14

Typeset in Bembo
Designed by Jaye Zimet with Joost Elffers
Printed and bound in Italy by
Legoprint S.p.a.—Lavis (TN)

The moral right of the author has been asserted.

All rights reserved. Without limiting the rights under copyright reserved above, no part of this publication may be reproduced, stored or introduced into a retrieval system, or transmitted, in any form or by any means (electronic, mechanical, photocopying, recording or otherwise), without the prior written permission of both the copyright owner and the publisher of this book.

A CIP catalogue record for this book is available from the British Library.

ISBN-10: 1 86197 641 0
ISBN-13: 978 1 86197 641 3

To the memory of my father

Grateful acknowledgment is made for permission to reprint excerpts from the following copyrighted works:

Falling in Love by Francesco Alberoni, translated by Lawrence Venuti. Reprinted by permission of Random House, Inc. *Seduction* by Jean Baudrillard, translated by Brian Singer, St. Martin's Press, 1990. Copyright © New World Perspectives, 1990. Reprinted by permission of Palgrave. *Warhol* by David Bourdon, published by Harry N. Abrams, Inc., New York. All rights reserved. Reprinted by permission of the publisher. *Andreas Capellanus on Love* by Andreas Capellanus, translated by P. G. Walsh. Reprinted by permission of Gerald Duckworth & Co. Ltd. *Portrait of a Seductress: The World of Natalie Barney* by Jean Chalon, translated by Carol Barko, Crown Publishers, Inc., 1979. Reprinted with permission. *Pursuit of the Millennium* by Norman Cohn. Copyright © 1970 by Oxford University Press. Used by permission of Oxford University Press, Inc. *Evita: The Real Life of Eva Peron* by Nicolas Fraser and Marysa Navarro, W. W. Norton & Company, Inc., 1996. Reprinted by permission. *The Greek Myths* by Robert Graves. Reprinted by permission of Carcanet Press Limited. *The Kennedy Obsession: The American Myth of JFK* by John Hellman, Columbia University Press, 1997. Reprinted by permission of Columbia University Press. *The Odyssey* by Homer, translated by E.V. Rieu (Penguin Classics, 1946). Copyright © The Estate of E.V. Rieu, 1946. Reprinted by permission of Penguin Books Ltd. *The Life of an Amorous Woman and Other Writings* by Ihara Saikaku, translated by Ivan Morris. Copyright © 1963 by New Directions Publishing Corp. Reprinted by permission of New Directions Publishing Corp. "The Seducer's Diary" from *Either/Or, Part 1* by Søren Kierkegaard, translated by Howard V. Hong and Edna H. Hong. Copyright © 1987 by

Princeton University Press. Reprinted by permission of Princeton University Press. *Don Juan and the Point of Horror* by James Mandrell. Reprinted with permission of Penn State University Press. *The Arts and Secrets of Beauty* by Lola Montez, Chelsea House, 1969. Used with permission. *The Age of the Crowd* by Serge Moscovici. Reprinted with permission of Cambridge University Press. *The Tale of Genji* by Murasaki Shikibu, translated by Edward G. Seidensticker, Alfred A. Knopf, 1976. Copyright © 1976 by Edward G. Seidensticker. Reprinted by permission of the publisher. *The Erotic Poems* by Ovid, translated by Peter Green (Penguin Classics, 1982). Copyright © Peter Green, 1982. Reprinted by permission of Penguin Books Ltd. *The Symposium* by Plato, translated by Walter Hamilton (Penguin Classics, 1951). Copyright © Walter Hamilton, 1951. Reprinted by permission of Penguin Books Ltd. *The Rise and Fall of Athens: Nine Greek Lives* by Plutarch, translated by Ian Scott-Kilvert (Penguin Classics, 1960). Copyright © Ian Scott-Kilvert, 1960. Reprinted by permission of Penguin Books Ltd. *Love Declared* by Denis de Rougemont, translated by Richard Howard. Reprinted by permission of Random House, Inc. *The Wisdom of Life and Counsels and Maxims* by Arthur Schopenhauer, translated by T. Bailey Saunders (Amherst, NY: Prometheus Books, 1995). Reprinted by permission of the publisher. *Liaison* by Joyce Wadler, published by Bantam Books, 1993. Reprinted by permission of the author. *Max Weber: Essays in Sociology* by Max Weber, edited and translated by H. H. Gerth and C. Wright Mills. Copyright 1946, 1958 by H. H. Gerth and C. Wright Mills. Used by permission of Oxford University Press, Inc. *The Game of Hearts: Harriette Wilson & Her Memoirs* edited by Lesley Blanch. Copyright © 1955 by Lesley Blanch. Reprinted with permission of Simon & Schuster.

Acknowledgments

First, I would like to thank Anna Biller for her countless contributions to this book: the research, the many discussions, her invaluable help with the text itself, and, last but not least, her knowledge of the art of seduction, of which I have been the happy victim on numerous occasions.

I must thank my mother, Laurette, for supporting me so steadfastly throughout this project and for being my most devoted fan.

I would like to thank Catherine Léouzon, who some years ago introduced me to *Les Liaisons Dangereuses* and the world of Valmont.

I would like to thank David Frankel, for his deft editing and for his much-appreciated advice; Molly Stern at Viking Penguin, for overseeing the project and helping to shape it; Radha Pancham, for keeping it all organized and being so patient; and Brett Kelly, for moving things along.

With heavy heart I would like to pay tribute to my cat Boris, who for thirteen years watched over me as I wrote and whose presence is sorely missed. His successor, Brutus, has proven to be a worthy muse.

Finally, I would like to honor my father. Words cannot express how much I miss him and how much he has inspired my work.

Contents

Preface • xi

Part One
The Seductive Character page 1

The Siren *page 5*
The Rake *page 11*
The Ideal Lover *page 16*
The Dandy *page 21*
The Natural *page 28*
The Coquette *page 34*
The Charmer *page 38*
The Charismatic *page 43*
The Star *page 51*

Part Two
The Seductive Process page 57

1 Choose the Right Victim *page 61*
2 Create a False Sense of Security—Approach Indirectly *page 65*
3 Send Mixed Signals *page 70*
4 Appear to Be an Object of Desire—Create Triangles *page 76*
5 Create a Need—Stir Anxiety and Discontent *page 82*
6 Master the Art of Insinuation *page 88*
7 Enter Their Spirit *page 93*
8 Create Temptation *page 97*
9 Keep Them in Suspense—What Comes Next? *page 103*

10 Use the Demonic Power of Words to Sow Confusion
page 108
11 Pay Attention to Detail   *page 115*
12 Poeticize Your Presence   *page 121*
13 Disarm Through Strategic Weakness and Vulnerability
page 126
14 Confuse Desire and Reality—The Perfect Illusion
page 131
15 Isolate the Victim   *page 137*
16 Prove Yourself   *page 143*
17 Effect a Regression   *page 149*
18 Stir Up the Transgressive and Taboo   *page 155*
19 Use Spiritual Lures   *page 161*
20 Mix Pleasure with Pain   *page 167*
21 Give Them Space to Fall—The Pursuer Is Pursued
page 174
22 Use Physical Lures   *page 182*
23 Master the Art of the Bold Move   *page 189*
24 Beware the Aftereffects   *page 196*

Selected Bibliography • 205

Preface

People are constantly trying to influence us, to tell us what to do, and just as often we tune them out, resisting their attempts at persuasion. There is a moment in our lives, however, when we all act differently—when we are in love. We fall under a kind of spell. Our minds are usually preoccupied with our own concerns; now they become filled with thoughts of the loved one. We grow emotional, lose the ability to think straight, act in foolish ways that we would never do otherwise. If this goes on long enough something inside us gives way: we surrender to the will of the loved one, and to our desire to possess them.

Seducers are people who understand the tremendous power contained in such moments of surrender. They analyze what happens when people are in love, study the psychological components of the process—what spurs the imagination, what casts a spell. By instinct and through practice they master the art of making people fall in love. As all great seducers know, it is much more effective to create love than lust. A person in love is emotional, pliable, and

> *Much more genius is needed to make love than to command armies.*
>
> —Ninon de L'Enclos

> *The first thing to get in your head is that every single / Girl can be caught—and that you'll catch her if / You set your toils right. Birds will sooner fall dumb in / Springtime, Cicadas in summer, or a hunting-dog / Turn his back on a hare, than a lover's bland inducements / Can fail with a woman. Even one you suppose / Reluctant will want it.*
>
> —Ovid, *The Art of Love*, translated by Peter Green

> *The combination of these two elements, enchantment and surrender, is, then, essential to the love which we are discussing ... What exists in love is surrender due to enchantment.*
>
> —José Ortega y Gasset, *On Love*, translated by Toby Talbot

easily misled. (The origin of the word "seduction" is the Latin for "to lead astray.") A person in lust is harder to control and, once satisfied, may easily leave you. Seducers take their time, create enchantment and the bonds of love, so that when sex ensues it only further enslaves the victim. Creating love and enchantment becomes the model for all seductions—sexual, social, political. A person in love will surrender.

It is pointless to try to argue against such power, to imagine that you are not interested in it, or that it is evil and ugly. The harder you try to resist the lure of seduction—as an idea, as a form of power—the more you will find yourself fascinated. The reason is simple: most of us have known the power of having someone fall in love with us. Our actions, gestures, the things we say, all have positive effects on this person; we may not completely understand what we have done right, but this feeling of power is intoxicating. It gives us confidence, which makes us more seductive. We may also experience this in a social or work setting—one day, we are in an elevated mood and people seem more responsive, more charmed by us. These moments of power are fleeting, but they resonate in the memory with great intensity. We want them back. The siren call of seduction is irresistible because power is irresistible, and nothing will bring you more power in the modern world than the ability to seduce.

To have such power does not require a total transformation in your character or any kind of physical improvement in your looks. Seduction is a game of psychology, not beauty, and it is within the grasp of any person to become a master at the game. All that is required is that you look at the world differently, through the eyes of a seducer.

Seducers are never self-absorbed. Their gaze is directed outward, not inward. When they meet someone their first move is to get inside that person's skin, to see the world through their eyes. Self-absorption is a sign of insecurity; it is anti-seductive. Everyone has insecurities, but seducers manage to ignore them, finding therapy for moments of self-doubt by being absorbed in the world. This gives them a buoyant spirit—we want to be around them. Getting into someone's skin, imagining what it is like to be them, helps the seducer gather valuable information, learn what makes that person tick, what will make them lose their ability to think straight and fall into a trap.

Seducers see themselves as providers of pleasure. As children we mostly devoted our lives to play and pleasure. Adults often have feelings of being cut off from this paradise,

> *What is good?— All that heightens the feeling of power, the will to power, power itself in man. • What is bad?—All that proceeds from weakness. • What is happiness?— The feeling that power increases— that a resistance is overcome.*
>
> —FRIEDRICH NIETZSCHE, THE ANTI-CHRIST, TRANSLATED BY R. J. HOLLINGDALE

of being weighed down by responsibilities. The seducer knows that people are waiting for pleasure—they never get enough of it from friends and lovers, and they cannot get it by themselves. A person who enters their lives offering adventure and romance cannot be resisted.

A seducer sees all of life as theater, everyone an actor. Most people feel they have constricted roles in life, which makes them unhappy. Seducers, on the other hand, can be anyone and can assume many roles. They take pleasure in performing. This freedom of theirs, this fluidity in body and spirit, is what makes them attractive.

The Art of Seduction is designed to arm you with weapons of persuasion and charm, so that those around you will slowly lose their ability to resist without knowing how or why it has happened.

Every seduction has two elements that you must analyze and understand: first, yourself and what is seductive about you; and second, your target and the actions that will penetrate their defenses and create surrender. The two sides are equally important. If you strategize without paying attention to the parts of your character that draw people to you, you will be seen as a mechanical seducer, slimy and manipulative. If you rely on your seductive personality without paying attention to the other person, you will make terrible mistakes and limit your potential.

Consequently, *The Art of Seduction* is divided into two parts. The first half, "The Seductive Character," describes the nine types of seducer. Studying these types will make you aware of what is inherently seductive in your character, the basic building block of any seduction. The second half, "The Seductive Process," includes the twenty-four maneuvers and strategies that will instruct you on how to create a spell, break down people's resistance, give movement and force to your seduction, and induce surrender in your target.

Once you enter these pages, let yourself be lured by the ideas, your mind open and your thoughts fluid. Slowly you will find yourself absorbing the poison through the skin and you will begin to see everything as a seduction, including the way you think and how you look at the world.

> *Most virtue is a demand for greater seduction.*
> —NATALIE BARNEY

Whatever is done from love always occurs beyond good and evil.

—FRIEDRICH NIETZSCHE, BEYOND GOOD AND EVIL, TRANSLATED BY WALTER KAUFMANN

Should anyone here in Rome lack finesse at love-making, \ Let him \ Try me—read my book, and results are guaranteed! \ Technique is the secret. Charioteer, sailor, oarsman, \ All need it. Technique can control \ Love himself.

—OVID, THE ART OF LOVE, TRANSLATED BY PETER GREEN

Part One
the Seductive Character

We all have the power of attraction—the ability to draw people in and hold them in our thrall. Far from all of us, though, are aware of this inner potential, and we imagine attractiveness instead as a near-mystical trait that a select few are born with and the rest will never command. Yet all we need to do to realize our potential is understand what it is in a person's character that naturally excites people and develop these latent qualities within us.

Successful seductions rarely begin with an obvious maneuver or strategic device. That is certain to arouse suspicion. Successful seductions begin with your character, your ability to radiate some quality that attracts people and stirs their emotions in a way that is beyond their control. Hypnotized by your seductive character, your victims will not notice your subsequent manipulations. It will then be child's play to mislead and seduce them.

There are nine seducer types in the world. Each type has a particular character trait that comes from deep within and creates a seductive pull. *Sirens* have an abundance of sexual energy and know how to use it. *Rakes* insatiably adore the opposite sex, and their desire is infectious. *Ideal Lovers* have an aesthetic sensibility that they apply to romance. *Dandies* like to play with their image, creating a striking and androgynous allure. *Naturals* are spontaneous and open. *Coquettes* are self-sufficient, with a fascinating cool at their core. *Charmers* want and know how to please—they are social creatures. *Charismatics* have an unusual confidence in themselves. *Stars* are ethereal and envelop themselves in mystery.

The chapters in this section will take you inside each of the nine types. At least one of the chapters should strike a chord—you will recognize part of yourself. That chapter will be the key to developing your own powers of attraction.

Think of the nine types as shadows, silhouettes. Only by stepping into one of them and letting it grow inside you can you begin to develop the seductive character that will bring you limitless power.

the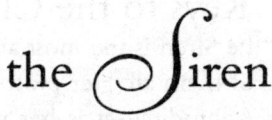

A man is often secretly oppressed by the role he has to play—by always having to be responsible, in control, and rational. The Siren is the ultimate male fantasy figure because she offers a total release from the limitations of his life. In her presence, which is always heightened and sexually charged, the male feels transported to a world of pure pleasure. She is dangerous, and in pursuing her energetically the man can lose control over himself, something he yearns to do. The Siren is a mirage; she lures men by cultivating a particular appearance and manner. In a world where women are often too timid to project such an image, learn to take control of the male libido by embodying his fantasy.

> *The charm of [Cleopatra's] presence was irresistible, and there was an attraction in her person and talk, together with a peculiar force of character, which pervaded her every word and action, and laid all who associated with her under its spell. It was a delight merely to hear the sound of her voice, with which, like an instrument of many strings, she could pass from one language to another.*
>
> —Plutarch,
> Makers of Rome,
> translated by Ian
> Scott-Kilvert

Keys to the Character

The Siren is the most ancient seductress of them all. Her prototype is the goddess Aphrodite—it is her nature to have a mythic quality about her—but do not imagine she is a thing of the past, or of legend and history: she represents a powerful male fantasy of a highly sexual, supremely confident, alluring female offering endless pleasure and a bit of danger. In today's world this fantasy can only appeal the more strongly to the male psyche, for now more than ever he lives in a world that circumscribes his aggressive instincts by making everything safe and secure, a world that offers less chance for adventure and risk than ever before. In the past, a man had some outlets for these drives—warfare, the high seas, political intrigue. In the sexual realm, courtesans and mistresses were practically a social institution, and offered him the variety and the chase that he craved. Without any outlets, his drives turn inward and gnaw at him, becoming all the more volatile for being repressed. Sometimes a powerful man will do the most irrational things, have an affair when it is least called for, just for a thrill, the danger of it all. The irrational can prove immensely seductive, even more so for men, who must always seem so reasonable.

If it is seductive power you are after, the Siren is the most potent of all. She operates on a man's most basic emotions, and if she plays her role properly, she can transform a normally strong and responsible male into a childish slave.

First and foremost, a Siren must distinguish herself from other women. She is by nature a rare thing, mythic, only one to a group; she is also a valuable prize to be wrested away from other men. Physicality offers the best opportunities here, since a Siren is preeminently a sight to behold. A highly feminine and sexual presence, even to the point of caricature, will quickly differentiate you, since most women lack the confidence to project such an image.

Once the Siren has made herself stand out from others, she must have two other critical qualities: the ability to get the male to pursue her so feverishly that he loses control; and a touch of the dangerous. Danger is surprisingly seductive. To get the male to pursue you is relatively simple: a highly sexual presence will do this quite well. But you must not resemble a courtesan or whore, whom the male may pursue only to quickly lose interest in her. Instead, you are slightly elusive and distant, a fantasy come to life. These qualities will make a man chase you vehemently, and the more

We're dazzled by feminine adornment, by the surface, \ All gold and jewels: so little of what we observe \ Is the girl herself. And where (you may ask) amid such plenty \ Can our object of passion be found? The eye's deceived \ By Love's smart camouflage.

—OVID, *CURES FOR LOVE*, TRANSLATED BY PETER GREEN

> *Your next encounter will be with the Sirens, who bewitch every man that approaches them ... For with the music of their song the Sirens cast their spell upon him, as they sit there in a meadow piled high with the moldering skeletons of men, whose withered skin still hangs upon their bones.*
>
> —CIRCE TO ODYSSEUS, *THE ODYSSEY*, BOOK XII

he chases, the more he will feel that he is acting on his own initiative.

An element of danger is easy to hint at, and will enhance your other Siren characteristics. Sirens are often fantastically irrational, which is immensely attractive to men who are oppressed by their own reasonableness. A touch of fear is also critical: it creates respect, keeping a man at a proper distance, so that he doesn't get close enough to see through you. Create such fear by suddenly changing your moods, keeping the man off balance, occasionally intimidating him with capricious behavior.

The most important element for an aspiring Siren is always the physical, the Siren's main instrument of power. Physical qualities—a scent, a heightened femininity evoked through makeup or through elaborate or seductive clothing—act all the more powerfully on men because they have no meaning. In their immediacy they bypass rational processes, having the same effect that a decoy has on an animal, or the movement of a cape on a bull. The proper Siren appearance is often confused with physical beauty, particularly the face. But a beautiful face does not a Siren make: instead it creates too much distance and coldness. The Siren must stimulate a generalized desire, and the best way to do this is by creating an overall impression that is both distracting and alluring. It is not one particular trait, but a combination of qualities:

The voice. Clearly a critical quality, as the legend indicates, the Siren's voice has an immediate animal presence with incredible suggestive power. The Siren must have an insinuating voice that hints at the erotic, more often subliminally than overtly. The Siren never speaks quickly, aggressively, or at a high pitch. Her voice is calm and unhurried, as if she had never quite woken up—or left her bed.

Body and adornment. If the voice must lull, the body and its adornment must dazzle. It is with her clothes that the Siren aims to create the goddess effect.

The key: everything must dazzle, but must also be harmonious, so that no single ornament draws attention. Your presence must be charged, larger than life, a fantasy come true. Ornament is used to cast a spell and distract. The Siren can also use clothing to hint at the sexual, at times overtly but more often by suggesting it rather than screaming it—that would make you seem manipulative. Related to this is the notion of selective disclosure, the revealing of only a part of the body—but a part that will excite and stir the imagination.

Movement and demeanor. The Siren moves gracefully and unhurriedly. The proper gestures, movement, and demeanor for a Siren are like the proper voice: they hint at something exciting, stirring desire without being obvious. Your air must be languorous, as if you had all the time in the world for love and pleasure. Your gestures must have a certain ambiguity, suggesting something both innocent and erotic, a perversely satisfying mix. While one part of you seems to scream sex, the other part is coy and naïve, as if you were incapable of understanding the effect you are having.

Symbol: *Water. The song of the Siren is liquid and enticing, and the Siren herself is fluid and ungraspable. Like the sea, the Siren lures you with the promise of infinite adventure and pleasure. Forgetting past and future, men follow her far out to sea, where they drown.*

the Rake

A woman never quite feels desired and appreciated enough. She wants attention, but a man is too often distracted and unresponsive. The Rake is a great female fantasy figure—when he desires a woman, brief though that moment may be, he will go to the ends of the earth for her. He may be disloyal, dishonest, and amoral, but that only adds to his appeal. Unlike the normal, cautious male, the Rake is delightfully unrestrained, a slave to his love of women. There is the added lure of his reputation: so many women have succumbed to him, there has to be a reason. Words are a woman's weakness, and the Rake is a master of seductive language. Stir a woman's repressed longings by adapting the Rake's mix of danger and pleasure.

Keys to the Character

> But what is this force, then, by which Don Juan seduces? It is desire, the energy of sensuous desire. He desires in every woman the whole of womanhood. The reaction to this gigantic passion beautifies and develops the one desired, who flushes in enhanced beauty by his reflection. As the enthusiast's fire with seductive splendor illumines even those who stand in a casual relation to him, so Don Juan transfigures in a far deeper sense every girl.
>
> —SØREN KIERKEGAARD, *EITHER/OR*

At first it may seem strange that a man who is clearly dishonest, disloyal, and has no interest in marriage would have any appeal to a woman. But throughout all of history, and in all cultures, this type has had a fatal effect. What the Rake offers is what society normally does not allow women: an affair of pure pleasure, an exciting brush with danger. A woman is often deeply oppressed by the role she is expected to play. She is supposed to be the tender, civilizing force in society, and to want commitment and lifelong loyalty. But often her marriages and relationships give her not romance and devotion but routine and an endlessly distracted mate. It remains an abiding female fantasy to meet a man who gives totally of himself, who lives for her, even if only for a while.

To play the Rake, the most obvious requirement is the ability to let yourself go, to draw a woman into the kind of purely sensual moment in which past and future lose meaning. Intense desire has a distracting power on a woman, just as the Siren's physical presence does on a man. A woman is often defensive and can sense insincerity or calculation. But if she feels consumed by your attentions, and is confident you will do anything for her, she will notice nothing else about you, or will find a way to forgive your indiscretions. The key is to show no hesitation, to abandon all restraint, to show that you cannot control yourself. Do not worry about inspiring mistrust; as long as you are the slave to her charms, she will not think of the aftermath.

The Rake never worries about a woman's resistance to him, or for that matter about any other obstacle in his path—a husband, a physical barrier. Resistance is only the spur to his desire, enflaming him all the more. Remember: if no resistances or obstacles face you, you must create them. No seduction can proceed without them.

Related to the Rake's extremism is the sense of danger, taboo, perhaps even the hint of cruelty about him. Just as a man may fall victim to the Siren through his desire to be free of his sense of masculine responsibility, a woman may succumb to the Rake through her yearning to be free of the constraints of virtue and decency. Indeed it is often the most virtuous woman who falls most deeply in love with the Rake. Like men, women are deeply attracted to the forbidden, the dangerous, even the slightly evil. Always remember: if you are to play the Rake, you must convey a sense of risk and darkness, suggesting to your victim that she is participating in

Among the many modes of handling Don Juan's effect on women, the motif of the irresistible hero is worth singling out, for it illustrates a curious change in our sensibility. Don Juan did not become irresistible to women until the Romantic age, and I am disposed to think that it is a trait of the female imagination to make him so. When the female voice began to assert itself and even, perhaps, to dominate in literature, Don Juan evolved to become the women's rather than the man's ideal ... Don Juan is now the woman's dream of the perfect lover, fugitive, passionate, daring. He gives her the one something rare and thrilling—a chance to play out her own rakish desires.

Among the Rake's most seductive qualities is his ability to make women want to reform him. You must exploit this tendency to the fullest. When caught red-handed in rakishness, fall back on your weakness—your desire to change, and your inability to do so. With so many women at your feet, what can you do? You are the one who is the victim. You need help. Women will jump at this opportunity; they are uncommonly indulgent of the Rake, for he is such a pleasant, dashing figure. The desire to reform him disguises the true nature of their desire, the secret thrill they get from him.

Each gender has its own weakness. The male is traditionally vulnerable to the visual. For women the weakness is language and words. The Rake must be as promiscuous with words as he is with women. He chooses words for their ability to suggest, insinuate, hypnotize, elevate, infect. The Rake's use of language is designed not to communicate or convey information but to persuade, flatter, stir emotional turmoil. Remember: it is the form that matters, not the content. Give your words a lofty, spiritual, literary flavor the better to insinuate desire.

Finally, a Rake's greatest asset is his reputation. Never downplay your bad name, or seem to apologize for it. Instead, embrace it, enhance it. It is what draws women to you. Do not leave your reputation to chance or gossip; it is your life's artwork, and you must craft it, hone it, and display it with the care of an artist.

Symbol:

Fire. The Rake burns with a desire that enflames the woman he is seducing. It is extreme, uncontrollable, and dangerous. The Rake may end in hell, but the flames surrounding him often make him seem that much more desirable to women.

unforgettable moment, the magnificent exaltation of the flesh which is too often denied her by the real husband, who thinks that men are gross and women spiritual. To be the fatal Don Juan may be the dream of a few men; but to meet him is the dream of many women.

—Oscar Mandel, "The Legend of Don Juan," in *The Theatre of Don Juan*, edited by Mandel

the Ideal lover

Most people have dreams in their youth that get shattered or worn down with age. They find themselves disappointed by people, events, reality, which cannot match their youthful ideals. Ideal Lovers thrive on people's broken dreams, which become lifelong fantasies. You long for romance? Adventure? Lofty spiritual communion? The Ideal Lover reflects your fantasy. He or she is an artist in creating the illusion you require, idealizing your portrait. In a world of disenchantment and baseness, there is limitless seductive power in following the path of the Ideal Lover.

Keys to the Character

Each of us carries inside us an ideal, either of what we would like to become, or of what we want another person to be for us. This ideal goes back to our earliest years—to what we once felt was missing in our lives, what others did not give to us, what we could not give to ourselves. Maybe we were smothered in comfort, and we long for danger and rebellion. If we want danger but it frightens us, perhaps we look for someone who seems at home with it. Or perhaps our ideal is more elevated—we want to be more creative, nobler, and kinder than we ever manage to be. Our ideal is something we feel is missing inside us.

Our ideal may be buried in disappointment, but it lurks underneath, waiting to be sparked. If another person seems to have that ideal quality, or to have the ability to bring it out in us, we fall in love. That is the response to Ideal Lovers. Attuned to what is missing inside you, to the fantasy that will stir you, they reflect your ideal—and you do the rest, projecting on to them your deepest desires and yearnings.

The Ideal Lover is rare in the modern world, for the role takes effort. You will have to focus intensely on the other person, fathom what she is missing, what he is disappointed by. People will often reveal

A good lover will behave as elegantly at dawn as at any other time. He drags himself out of bed with a look of dismay on his face. The lady urges him on: "Come, my friend, it's getting light. You don't want anyone to find you here." He gives a deep sigh, as if to say that the night has not been nearly long enough and that it is agony to leave. Once up, he does not instantly pull on his trousers. Instead he comes close to the lady and whispers whatever was left unsaid during the night. Even when he is dressed, he still lingers, vaguely pretending to be fastening his sash. Presently he raises the lattice, and the two lovers stand

this in subtle ways. Ignore your targets' words and conscious behavior; focus on the tone of their voice, a blush here, a look there—those signs that betray what their words won't say. By seeming to be what they lack, you will fit their ideal.

To create this effect requires patience and attention to detail. Most people are so wrapped up in their own desires, so impatient, they are incapable of the Ideal Lover role. Let that be a source of infinite opportunity. Be like an oasis in the desert of the self-absorbed; few can resist the temptation of following a person who seems so attuned to their desires, to bringing to life their fantasies.

The embodiment of the Ideal Lover for the 1920s was Rudolph Valentino, or at least the image created of him in film. Everything he did—the gifts, the flowers, the dancing, the way he took a woman's hand—showed a scrupulous attention to the details that would signify how much he was thinking of her. The image was of a man who made courtship take time, transforming it into an aesthetic experience. Men hated Valentino, because women now expected them to match the ideal of patience and attentiveness that he represented. Yet nothing is more seductive than patient attentiveness. It makes the affair seem lofty, aesthetic, not really about sex. The power of a Valentino, particularly nowadays, is that people like this are so rare. The art of playing to a woman's ideal has almost disappeared—which only makes it that much more alluring.

If the chivalrous lover remains the ideal for women, men often idealize the Madonna/whore, a woman who combines sensuality with an air of spirituality or innocence. The key is ambiguity—to combine the appearance of sensitivity to the pleasures of the flesh with an air of innocence, spirituality, a poetic sensibility. This mix of the high and the low is immensely seductive.

If Ideal Lovers are masters at seducing people by appealing to their higher selves, to something lost from their childhood, politicians can benefit by applying this skill on a mass scale, to an entire electorate. This was what John F. Kennedy quite deliberately did with the American public, most obviously in creating the "Camelot" aura around himself. The word "Camelot" was applied to his presidency only after his death, but the romance he consciously projected through his youth and good looks was fully functioning during his lifetime. More subtly, he also played with America's images of its own greatness and lost ideals. People literally fell in love with him and the image.

> *together by the side door while he tells her how he dreads the coming day, which will keep them apart; then he slips away. The lady watches him go, and this moment of parting will remain among her most charming memories. Indeed, one's attachment to a man depends largely on the elegance of his leave-taking. When he jumps out of bed, scurries about the room, tightly fastens his trouser sash, rolls up the sleeves of his court cloak ... stuffs his belongings into the breast of his robe and then briskly secures the outer sash—one really begins to hate him.*
>
> —THE PILLOW BOOK OF SEI SHONAGON, TRANSLATED AND EDITED BY IVAN MORRIS

> *Women have served all these centuries as looking glasses possessing the magic and delicious power of reflecting the figure of a man at twice its natural size.*
>
> —VIRGINIA WOOLF, *A ROOM OF ONE'S OWN*

Remember: most people believe themselves to be inwardly greater than they outwardly appear to the world. They are full of unrealized ideals: they could be artists, thinkers, leaders, spiritual figures, but the world has crushed them, denied them the chance to let their abilities flourish. This is the key to their seduction—and to keeping them seduced over time. Appeal only to people's physical side, as many amateur seducers do, and they will resent you for playing upon their basest instincts. But appeal to their better selves, to a higher standard of beauty, and they will hardly notice that they have been seduced. Make them feel elevated, lofty, spiritual, and your power over them will be limitless.

***Symbol:** The Portrait Painter. Under his eye, all of your physical imperfections disappear. He brings out noble qualities in you, frames you in a myth, makes you godlike, immortalizes you. For his ability to create such fantasies, he is rewarded with great power.*

the *Dandy*

*Most
of us feel trapped within
the limited roles that the world expects us to play. We are instantly attracted
to those who are more fluid, more ambiguous,
than we are—those who create their own persona.
Dandies excite us because they cannot be categorized, and hint at a freedom we want for ourselves.
They play with masculinity and femininity; they fashion their own physical image, which is always startling;
they are mysterious and elusive. They also appeal to
the narcissism of each sex: to a woman they are psychologically female, to a man they are male.
Dandies fascinate and seduce in large numbers.
Use the power of the Dandy to create an
ambiguous, alluring presence that
stirs repressed desires.*

Keys to the Character

*Dandyism is not even, as many unthinking people seem to suppose, an immoderate interest in personal appearance and material elegance. For the true dandy these things are only a symbol of the aristocratic superiority of his personality ...
• What, then, is this ruling passion that has turned into a creed and created its own skilled tyrants? What is this unwritten constitution that has created so haughty a caste? It is, above all, a burning need to acquire originality, within the apparent bounds of convention. It is a sort of cult of oneself, which can dispense even with what are commonly called illusions. It is the delight in causing astonishment, and the proud*

Many of us today imagine that sexual freedom has progressed in recent years—that everything has changed, for better or worse. This is mostly an illusion; a reading of history reveals periods of licentiousness (imperial Rome, late-seventeenth-century England, the "floating world" of eighteenth-century Japan) far in excess of what we are currently experiencing. Gender roles are certainly changing, but they have changed before. Society is in a state of constant flux, but there is something that does not change: the vast majority of people conform to whatever is normal for the time. They play the role allotted to them. Conformity is a constant because humans are social creatures who are always imitating one another.

Dandies have existed in all ages and cultures and wherever they have gone they have thrived on the conformist role playing of others. The Dandy displays a true and radical difference from other people, a difference of appearance and manner. Since most of us are secretly oppressed by our lack of freedom, we are drawn to those who are more fluid and flaunt their difference.

Dandies seduce socially as well as sexually; groups form around them, their style is wildly imitated, an entire court or crowd will fall in love with them. In adapting the Dandy character for your own purposes, remember that the Dandy is by nature a rare and beautiful flower. Be different in ways that are both striking and aesthetic, never vulgar; poke fun at current trends and styles, go in a novel direction, and be supremely uninterested in what anyone else is doing. Most people are insecure; they will wonder what you are up to, and slowly they will come to admire and imitate you, because you express yourself with total confidence.

The Dandy has traditionally been defined by clothing, and certainly most Dandies create a unique visual style. Beau Brummel, the most famous Dandy of all, would spend hours on his toilette, particularly the inimitably styled knot in his necktie, for which he was famous throughout early-nineteenth-century England. But a Dandy's style cannot be obvious, for Dandies are subtle, and never try hard for attention—attention comes to them. The person whose clothes are flagrantly different has little imagination or taste. Dandies show their difference in the little touches that mark their disdain for convention: Oscar Wilde's green velvet suit, Andy Warhol's silver wigs. The female Dandy works similarly. She may adopt male clothing, say, but if she

satisfaction of never oneself being astonished ...

—CHARLES BAUDELAIRE, *THE DANDY*, QUOTED IN *VICE: AN ANTHOLOGY*, EDITED BY RICHARD DAVENPORT-HINES

> *I am a woman. Every artist is a woman and should have a taste for other women. Artists who are homosexual cannot be true artists because they like men, and since they themselves are women they are reverting to normality.*
>
> —Pablo Picasso

does, a touch here or there will set her truly apart: no man ever dressed quite like George Sand. The overtall hat, the riding boots worn on the streets of Paris, made her a sight to behold.

Remember, there must be a reference point. If your visual style is totally unfamiliar, people will think you at best an obvious attention-getter, at worst crazy. Instead, create your own fashion sense by adapting and altering prevailing styles to make yourself an object of fascination. Do this right and you will be wildly imitated.

The nonconformity of Dandies, however, goes far beyond appearances. It is an attitude toward life that sets them apart; adopt that attitude and a circle of followers will form around you.

Dandies are supremely impudent. They don't give a damn about other people, and never try to please. The insolence of the Dandy is aimed at society and its conventions. And since people are generally oppressed by the obligation of always being polite and self-sacrificing, they are delighted to spend time around a person who disdains such niceties.

Dandies are masters of the art of living. They live for pleasure, not for work; they surround themselves with beautiful objects and eat and drink with the same relish they show for their clothes. The key is to make everything an aesthetic choice. Your ability to alleviate boredom by making life an art will make your company highly prized.

The opposite sex is a strange country we can never know, and this excites us, creates the proper sexual tension. But it is also a source of annoyance and frustration. Men do not understand how women think, and vice versa; each tries to make the other act more like a member of their own sex. Dandies may never try to please, but in this one area they have a pleasing effect: by adopting psychological traits of the opposite sex, they appeal to our inherent narcissism. This kind of mental transvestism—the ability to enter the spirit of the opposite sex, adapt to their way of thinking, mirror their tastes and attitudes—can be a key element in seduction. It is a way of mesmerizing your victim.

The Feminine Dandy (the slightly androgynous male) lures the woman in with exactly what she wants—a familiar, pleasing, graceful presence. Mirroring feminine psychology, he displays attention to his appearance, sensitivity to detail, a slight coquettishness—but also a hint of male cruelty. Women are narcissists, in love with the charms of their own sex. By showing them feminine charm, a man can mesmerize and

> *This royal manner which [the dandy] raises to the height of true royalty, the dandy has taken this from women, who alone seem naturally made for such a role. It is a somewhat by using the manner and the method of women that the dandy dominates. And this usurpation of femininity, he makes women themselves approve of this ... The dandy has something antinatural and androgynous about him, which is precisely how he is able to endlessly seduce.*
>
> —JULES LEMAÎTRE, LES CONTEMPORAINS

disarm them, leaving them vulnerable to a bold, masculine move.

The Masculine Dandy (the slightly androgynous female) succeeds by reversing the normal pattern of male superiority in matters of love and seduction. A man's apparent independence, his capacity for detachment, often seems to give him the upper hand in the dynamic between men and women. A purely feminine woman will arouse desire, but is always vulnerable to the man's capricious loss of interest; a purely masculine woman, on the other hand, will not arouse that interest at all. Follow the path of the Masculine Dandy, however, and you neutralize all a man's powers. Never give completely of yourself; while you are passionate and sexual, always retain an air of independence and self-possession. You might move on to the next man, or so he will think. You have other, more important matters to concern yourself with, such as your work. Men do not know how to fight women who use their own weapons against them; they are intrigued, aroused, and disarmed.

According to Freud, the human libido is essentially bisexual; most people are in some way attracted to people of their own sex, but social constraints (varying with culture and historical period) repress these impulses. The Dandy represents a release from such constraints.

Do not be misled by the surface disapproval your Dandy pose may elicit. Society may publicize its distrust of androgyny (in Christian theology, Satan is often represented as androgynous), but this conceals its fascination; what is most seductive is often what is most repressed. Learn a playful dandyism and you will become the magnet for people's dark, unrealized yearnings.

The key to such power is ambiguity. In a society where the roles everyone plays are obvious, the refusal to conform to any standard will excite interest. Be both masculine and feminine, impudent and charming, subtle and outrageous. Let other people worry about being socially acceptable; those types are a dime a dozen, and you are after a power greater than they can imagine.

Symbol: *The Orchid. Its shape and color oddly suggest both sexes, its odor is sweet and decadent—it is a tropical flower of evil. Delicate and highly cultivated, it is prized for its rarity; it is unlike any other flower.*

the Natural

*Child-
hood is the golden paradise
we are always consciously or unconsciously trying to re-create. The Natural
embodies the longed-for qualities of childhood—spontaneity, sincerity, unpretentiousness. In
the presence of Naturals, we feel at ease, caught up in
their playful spirit, transported back to that golden age.
Naturals also make a virtue out of weakness, eliciting
our sympathy for their trials, making us want to protect
them and help them. As with a child, much of this is
natural, but some of it is exaggerated, a conscious
seductive maneuver. Adopt the pose of the
Natural to neutralize people's natural
defensiveness and infect them with
helpless delight.*

Psychological Traits of the Natural

Children are not as guileless as we like to imagine. They suffer from feelings of helplessness, and sense early on the power of their natural charm to remedy their weakness in the adult world. They learn to play a game: if their natural innocence can persuade a parent to yield to their desires in one instance, then it is something they can use strategically in another instance, laying it on thick at the right moment to get their way. If their vulnerability and weakness is so attractive, then it is something they can use for effect.

A child represents a world from which we have been forever exiled. Because adult life is full of boredom and compromise, we harbor an illusion of childhood as a kind of golden age, even though it can often be a period of great confusion and pain. It cannot be denied, however, that childhood had certain privileges, and as children we had a pleasurable attitude to life. Confronted with a particularly charming child, we often feel wistful: we remember our own golden past, the qualities we have lost and wish we had again. And in the presence of the child, we get a little of that goldenness back.

Natural seducers are people who somehow avoided getting certain childish traits

Long-past ages have a great and often puzzling attraction for men's imagination. Whenever they are dissatisfied with their present surroundings—and this happens often enough—they turn back to the past and hope that they will now be able to prove the truth of the inextinguishable dream of a golden age. They are probably still under the spell of their childhood, which is presented to them by their not impartial memory as a time of uninterrupted bliss.

—SIGMUND FREUD, THE STANDARD EDITION OF THE COMPLETE PSYCHOLOGICAL WORKS OF SIGMUND FREUD, VOLUME 23

A man may meet a woman and be shocked by her ugliness. Soon, if she is natural and unaffected, her expression makes him overlook the fault of her features. He begins to find her charming, it enters his head that she might be loved, and a week later he is living in hope. The following week he has been snubbed into despair, and the week afterwards he has gone mad.

—Stendhal, *Love*, translated by Gilbert and Suzanne Sale

drummed out of them by adult experience. Such people can be as powerfully seductive as any child, because it seems uncanny and marvelous that they have preserved such qualities. They are not literally like children, of course; that would make them obnoxious or pitiful. Rather it is the spirit that they have retained. Do not imagine that this childishness is something beyond their control. Natural seducers learn early on the value of retaining a particular quality, and the seductive power it contains; they adapt and build upon those childlike traits that they managed to preserve, exactly as the child learns to play with its natural charm. This is the key. It is within your power to do the same, since there is lurking within all of us a devilish child straining to be let loose.

The following are the main types of the adult Natural. Keep in mind that the greatest natural seducers are often a blend of more than one of these qualities.

The innocent. The adult Natural is not truly innocent—it is impossible to grow up in this world and retain total innocence. Yet Naturals yearn so deeply to hold on to their innocent outlook that they manage to preserve the illusion of innocence. They exaggerate their weakness to elicit the proper sympathy. They act like they still see the world through innocent eyes, which in an adult proves doubly humorous. Much of this is conscious, but to be effective, adult Naturals must make it seem subtle and effortless—if they are seen as *trying* to act innocent, it will come across as pathetic. Learn to play up any natural weaknesses or flaws.

The imp. Impish children have a fearlessness that we adults have lost. That is because they do not see the possible consequences of their actions—how some people might be offended, how they might physically hurt themselves in the process. Imps are brazen, blissfully uncaring. They infect you with their lighthearted spirit. Such children have not yet had their natural energy and spirit scolded out of them by the need to be polite and civil. Secretly, we envy them; we want to be naughty too.

Adult imps are seductive because of how different they are from the rest of us. Breaths of fresh air in a cautious world, they go full throttle, as if their impishness were uncontrollable, and thus natural. If you play the part, do not worry about offending people now and then—you are too lovable and inevitably they will forgive you.

The wonder. A wonder child has a special, inexplicable talent: a gift for music, for mathematics, for chess, for sport. At work in the field in which they have such prodigal skill, these children seem possessed, and their actions effortless. If they are artists or musicians, Mozart types, their work seems to spring from some inborn impulse, requiring remarkably little thought. If it is a physical talent that they have, they are blessed with unusual energy, dexterity, and spontaneity. In both cases they seem talented beyond their years. This fascinates us.

Adult wonders are often former wonder children who have managed, remarkably, to retain their youthful impulsiveness and improvisational skills. To play the wonder you need some skill that seems easy and natural, along with the ability to improvise. If in fact your skill takes practice, you must hide this and learn to make your work appear effortless. The more you hide the sweat behind what you do, the more natural and seductive it will appear.

The undefensive lover. As people get older, they protect themselves against painful experiences by closing themselves off. The price for this is that they grow rigid, physically and mentally. But children are by nature unprotected and open to experience, and this receptiveness is extremely attractive. In the presence of children we become less rigid, infected with their openness. That is why we want to be around them.

Undefensive lovers have somehow circumvented the self-protective process, retaining the playful, receptive spirit of the child. The undefensive lover lowers the inhibitions of his or her target, a critical part of seduction. Be open to influence from others, and they will more easily fall under your spell.

Symbol: The Lamb.
So soft and endearing.
At two days old the lamb
can gambol gracefully; within
a week it is playing "Follow
the Leader." Its weakness is part
of its charm. The Lamb is pure
innocence, so innocent we want
to possess it, even devour it.

the Coquette

The ability to delay satisfaction is the ultimate art of seduction—while waiting, the victim is held in thrall. Coquettes are the grand masters of this game, orchestrating a back-and-forth movement between hope and frustration. They bait with the promise of reward—the hope of physical pleasure, happiness, fame by association, power—all of which, however, proves elusive; yet this only makes their targets pursue them the more. Coquettes seem totally self-sufficient: they do not need you, they seem to say, and their narcissism proves devilishly attractive. You want to conquer them but they hold the cards. The strategy of the Coquette is never to offer total satisfaction. Imitate the alternating heat and coolness of the Coquette and you will keep the seduced at your heels.

Keys to the Character

According to the popular concept, Coquettes are consummate teases, experts at arousing desire through a provocative appearance or an alluring attitude. But the real essence of Coquettes is in fact their ability to trap people emotionally, and to keep their victims in their clutches long after that first titillation of desire. This is the skill that puts them in the ranks of the most effective seducers.

To understand the peculiar power of the Coquette, you must first understand a critical property of love and desire: the more obviously you pursue a person, the more likely you are to chase them away. Too much attention can be interesting for a while, but it soon grows cloying and finally becomes claustrophobic and frightening. It signals weakness and neediness, an unseductive combination. How often we make this mistake, thinking our persistent presence will reassure. But Coquettes have an inherent understanding of this particular dynamic. Masters of selective withdrawal, they hint at coldness, absenting themselves at times to keep their victim off balance, surprised, intrigued. Their withdrawals make them mysterious, and we build them up in our imaginations. A bout of distance engages the emotions further; instead of making us

[Narcissistic] women have the greatest fascination for men ... The charm of a child lies to a great extent in his narcissism, his self-sufficiency and inaccessibility, just as does the charm of certain animals which seem not to concern themselves about us, such as cats ... It is as if we envied them their power of retaining a blissful state of mind—an unassailable libido-position which we ourselves have since abandoned.

—SIGMUND FREUD

> *Coquettes know how to please; not how to love, which is why men love them so much.*
>
> —PIERRE MARIVAUX

> *An absence, the declining of an invitation to dinner, an unintentional, unconscious harshness are of more service than all the cosmetics and fine clothes in the world.*
>
> —MARCEL PROUST

> *She who would long retain her power must use her lover ill.*
>
> —OVID

angry, it makes us insecure. Perhaps they don't really like us, perhaps we have lost their interest. Once our vanity is at stake, we succumb to the Coquette just to prove we are still desirable. Remember: the essence of the Coquette lies not in the tease and temptation but in the subsequent step back, the emotional withdrawal. That is the key to enslaving desire.

Coquettes are not emotionally needy; they are self-sufficient. And this is surprisingly seductive. Self-esteem is critical in seduction. Low self-esteem repels, confidence and self-sufficiency attract. The less you seem to need other people, the more likely others will be drawn to you. Understand the importance of this in all relationships and you will find your neediness easier to suppress.

The Coquette must first and foremost be able to excite the target of his or her attention. The attraction can be sexual, the lure of celebrity, whatever it takes. At the same time, the Coquette sends contrary signals that stimulate contrary responses, plunging the victim into confusion.

Coquetry depends on developing a pattern to keep the other person off balance. The strategy is extremely effective. Experiencing a pleasure once, we yearn to repeat it; so the Coquette gives us pleasure, then withdraws it.

Coquettes are never jealous—that would undermine their image of fundamental self-sufficiency. But they are masters at inciting jealousy: by paying attention to a third party, creating a triangle of desire, they signal to their victims that they may not be that interested. This triangulation is extremely seductive, in social contexts as well as erotic ones. Remember to keep an emotional and physical distance. This will allow you to cry and laugh on command, project self-sufficiency, and with such detachment you will be able play people's emotions like a piano.

Symbol: *The Shadow. It cannot be grasped. Chase your shadow and it will flee; turn your back on it and it will follow you. It is also a person's dark side, the thing that makes them mysterious. After they have given us pleasure, the shadow of their withdrawal makes us yearn for their return, much as clouds make us yearn for the sun.*

There is a way to represent one's cause and in doing so to treat the audience in such a cool and condescending manner that they are bound to notice one is not doing it to please them. The principle should always be not to make concessions to those who don't have anything to give but who have everything to gain from us. We can wait until they are begging on their knees even if it takes a very long time.

—SIGMUND FREUD, IN A LETTER TO A PUPIL, QUOTED IN PAUL ROAZEN, *FREUD AND HIS FOLLOWERS*

the *Charmer*

*Charm is seduction without sex. Charmers
are consummate manipulators, masking their clev-
erness by creating a mood of pleasure and comfort.
Their method is simple: they deflect attention from
themselves and focus it on their target. They understand
your spirit, feel your pain, adapt to your moods. In the
presence of a Charmer you feel better about yourself.
Charmers do not argue or fight, complain, or pester—
what could be more seductive? By drawing you in
with their indulgence they make you dependent
on them, and their power grows. Learn to cast
the Charmer's spell by aiming at people's
primary weaknesses: vanity and
self-esteem.*

The Art of Charm

Sexuality is extremely disruptive. The insecurities and emotions it stirs up can often cut short a relationship that would otherwise be deeper and longer lasting. The Charmer's solution is to fulfill the aspects of sexuality that are so alluring and addictive—the focused attention, the boosted self-esteem, the pleasurable wooing, the understanding (real or illusory)—but subtract the sex itself. It's not that the Charmer represses or discourages sexuality; lurking beneath the surface of any attempt at charm is a sexual tease, a possibility. Charm cannot exist without a hint of sexual tension. It cannot be maintained, however, unless sex is kept at bay or in the background.

The word "charm" comes from the Latin *carmen,* a song, but also an incantation tied to the casting of a magical spell. The Charmer implicitly grasps this history, casting a spell by giving people something that holds their attention, that fascinates them. And the secret to capturing people's attention, while lowering their powers of reason, is to strike at the thing they have the least control over: their ego, their vanity and self-esteem. As Benjamin Disraeli said, "Talk to a man about himself and he will listen for hours." The strategy can never be obvious; subtlety is the Charmer's great skill. If the

> *Birds are taken with pipes that imitate their own voices, and men with those sayings that are most agreeable to their own opinions.*
>
> —SAMUEL BUTLER

> *You know what charm is: a way of getting the answer yes without having asked any clear question.*
>
> —ALBERT CAMUS

> *Go with the bough, you'll bend it; / Use brute force, it'll snap. / Go with the current: that's how to swim across rivers— / Fighting upstream's no good. / Go easy with lions or tigers if you aim to tame them; / The bull gets inured to the plough by slow degrees ... / So, yield if she shows resistance: / That way you'll win in the end.*
>
> — OVID, *THE ART OF LOVE*, TRANSLATED BY PETER GREEN

target is to be kept from seeing through the Charmer's efforts, and from growing suspicious, maybe even tiring of the attention, a light touch is essential.

The following are the laws of charm.

Make your target the center of attention. Charmers fade into the background; their targets become the subject of their interest. To be a Charmer you have to learn to listen and observe. Let your targets talk, revealing themselves in the process. As you find out more about them, you can individualize your attention, appealing to their specific desires and needs, tailoring your flatteries to their insecurities. Make them the star of the show and they will become addicted to you and grow dependent on you.

Be a source of pleasure. No one wants to hear about your problems and troubles. Listen to your targets' complaints, but more important, distract them from their problems by giving them pleasure. (Do this often enough and they will fall under your spell.) Being lighthearted and fun is always more charming than being serious and critical.

Bring antagonism into harmony. Never stir up antagonisms that will prove immune to your charm; in the face of those who are aggressive, retreat, let them have their little victories. Yielding and indulgence will charm the fight out of any potential enemies. Never criticize people overtly—that will make them insecure, and resistant to change. Plant ideas, insinuate suggestions.

Lull your victims into ease and comfort. Charm is like the hypnotist's trick with the swinging watch: the more relaxed the target, the easier it is to bend him or her to your will. The key to making your victims feel comfortable is to mirror them, adapt to their moods. People are narcissists— they are drawn to those most similar to themselves. Seem to share their values and tastes, to understand their spirit, and they will fall under your spell.

Show calm and self-possession in the face of adversity. Adversity and setbacks actually provide the perfect setting for charm. Showing a calm, unruffled exterior in the face of unpleasantness puts people at ease. Never whine, never complain, never try to justify yourself.

Make yourself useful. If done subtly, your ability to enhance the lives of others will

A speech that carries its audience along with it and is applauded is often less suggestive simply because it is clear that it sets out to be persuasive. People talking together influence each other in close proximity by means of the tone of voice they adopt and the way they look at each other and not only by the kind of language they use. We are right to call a good conversationalist a charmer in the magical sense of the word.

—GUSTAVE TARDE, *L'OPINION ET LA FOULE*, QUOTED IN SERGE MOSCOVICI, *THE AGE OF THE CROWD* be devilishly seductive. Your social skills will prove important here: creating a wide network of allies will give you the power to link people up with each other, which will make them feel that by knowing you they can make their lives easier. This is something no one can resist. Follow-through is key. Anyone can make a promise; what sets you apart, and makes you charming, is your ability to come through in the end, following up your promise with a definite action.

Symbol: The Mirror. Your spirit holds a mirror up to others. When they see you they see themselves: their values, their tastes, even their flaws. Their lifelong love affair with their own image is comfortable and hypnotic; so feed it. No one ever sees what is behind the mirror.

the Charismatic

*Charisma
is a presence that excites us. It
comes from an inner quality—self-confidence, sexual energy, sense of purpose, contentment—that most people lack and want. This
quality radiates outward, permeating the gestures
of Charismatics, making them seem extraordinary
and superior, and making us imagine there is more
to them than meets the eye: they are gods, saints,
stars. Charismatics can learn to heighten their
charisma with a piercing gaze, fiery oratory,
an air of mystery. They can seduce on a
grand scale. Learn to create the
charismatic illusion by radiating
intensity while remain-
ing detached.*

> *"Charisma" shall be understood to refer to an extraordinary quality of a person, regardless of whether this quality is actual, alleged or presumed. "Charismatic authority," hence, shall refer to a rule over men, whether predominately external or predominately internal, to which the governed submit because of their belief in the extraordinary quality of the specific person.*
>
> —Max Weber, from *Max Weber: Essays in Sociology*, edited by Hans Gerth and C. Wright Mills

Charisma and Seduction

Charisma is seduction on a mass level. Charismatics make crowds of people fall in love with them, then lead them along. The process of making them fall in love is simple and follows a path similar to that of a one-on-one seduction. Charismatics have certain qualities that are powerfully attractive and that make them stand out. This could be their self-belief, their boldness, their serenity. They keep the source of these qualities mysterious. They do not explain where their confidence or contentment comes from, but it can be felt by everyone; it radiates outward, without the appearance of conscious effort. The face of the Charismatic is usually animated, full of energy, desire, alertness—the look of a lover, one that is instantly appealing, even vaguely sexual. We happily follow Charismatics because we like to be led, particularly by people who promise adventure or prosperity. We lose ourselves in their cause, become emotionally attached to them, feel more alive by believing in them—we fall in love.

Charisma plays on repressed sexuality, creates an erotic charge. Yet the origins of the word lie not in sexuality but in religion, and religion remains deeply embedded in modern charisma.

Thousands of years ago, people believed in gods and spirits, but few could ever say that they had witnessed a miracle, a physical demonstration of divine power. A man, however, who seemed possessed by a divine spirit—speaking in tongues, ecstatic raptures, the expression of intense visions—would stand out as one whom the gods had singled out. And this man, a priest or a prophet, gained great power over others. Most of the great religions were founded by a Charismatic, a person who physically displayed the signs of God's favor.

Today, anyone who has presence, who attracts attention when he or she enters a room, is said to possess charisma. But even these less-exalted types reveal a trace of the quality suggested by the word's original meaning. Their charisma is mysterious and inexplicable, never obvious. They have an unusual confidence. They have a gift—often a smoothness with language—that makes them stand out from the crowd. They express a vision.

Charisma must seem mystical, but that does not mean you cannot learn certain tricks that will enhance the charisma you already possess, or will give you the outward appearance of it. The following are basic qualities that will help create the illusion of charisma:

> *That devil of a man exercises a fascination on me that I cannot explain even to myself, and in such a degree that, though I fear neither God nor devil, when I am in his presence I am ready to tremble like a child, and he could make me go through the eye of a needle to throw myself into the fire.*
>
> —GENERAL VANDAMME, ON NAPOLEON BONAPARTE

> [The masses] have never thirsted after truth. They demand illusions, and cannot do without them. They constantly give what is unreal precedence over what is real; they are almost as strongly influenced by what is untrue as by what is true. They have an evident tendency not to distinguish between the two.
> —SIGMUND FREUD, THE STANDARD EDITION OF THE COMPLETE PSYCHOLOGICAL WORKS OF SIGMUND FREUD, VOLUME 18

Purpose. If people believe you have a plan, that you know where you are going, they will follow you instinctively. The direction does not matter: pick a cause, an ideal, a vision and show that you will not sway from your goal. People will imagine that your confidence comes from something real.

Mystery. Mystery lies at charisma's heart, but it is a particular kind of mystery—a mystery expressed by contradiction. The Charismatic may be both proletarian and aristocratic (Mao Zedong), both excitable and icily detached (Charles de Gaulle), both intimate and distant (Sigmund Freud). Since most people are predictable, the effect of these contradictions is devastatingly charismatic. They make you hard to fathom, add richness to your character, make people talk about you. Show your mysteriousness gradually and word will spread. You must also keep people at arm's length, to keep them from figuring you out.

Saintliness. Most of us must compromise constantly to survive; saints do not. They must live out their ideals without caring about the consequences. The saintly effect bestows charisma.

Saintliness goes far beyond religion: politicians as disparate as George Washington and Lenin won saintly reputations by living simply, despite their power—by matching their political values to their personal lives. Both men were virtually deified after they died. The key is that you must already have some deeply held values; that part cannot be faked, at least not without risking accusations of charlatanry that will destroy your charisma in the long run. The next step is to show, as simply and subtly as possible, that you live what you believe.

Eloquence. A Charismatic relies on the power of words. The reason is simple: words are the quickest way to create emotional disturbance. They can uplift, elevate, stir anger, without referring to anything real. Eloquence can be learned. Roosevelt, a calm, patrician type, was able to make himself a dynamic speaker, both through his style of delivery, which was slow and hypnotic, and through his brilliant use of imagery, alliteration, and biblical rhetoric. The slow, authoritative style is often more effective than passionate oratory, for it is more subtly spellbinding, and less tiring.

Theatricality. A Charismatic is larger than life, has extra presence. Actors have studied this kind of presence for centuries; they

Genuine charisma thus means the ability to internally generate and externally express extreme excitement, an ability which makes one the object of intense attention and unreflective imitation by others.

—LIAH GREENFIELD

know how to stand on a crowded stage and command attention. Surprisingly, it is not the actor who screams the loudest or gestures the most wildly who works this magic best, but the actor who stays calm, radiating self-assurance. The effect is ruined by trying too hard.

Uninhibitedness. Most people are repressed, and have little access to their unconscious—a problem that creates opportunities for the Charismatic, who can become a kind of screen on which others project their secret fantasies and longings. You will first have to show that you are less inhibited than your audience—that you radiate a dangerous sexuality, have no fear of death, are delightfully spontaneous. Even a hint of these qualities will make people think you more powerful than you are.

Fervency. You need to believe in something, and to believe in it strongly enough for it to animate all your gestures and make your eyes light up. A prerequisite for fiery belief is some great cause to rally around—a crusade. Become the rallying point for people's discontent, and show that you share none of the doubts that plague normal humans. People are more and more isolated, and long for communal experience. Let your own fervent and contagious faith, in virtually anything, give them something to believe in.

Vulnerability. Charismatics display a need for love and affection. They are open to their audience, and in fact feed off its energy; the audience in turn is electrified by the Charismatic, the current increasing as it passes back and forth. Since charisma involves feelings akin to love, you in turn must reveal your love for your followers. Imagine your public as a single person whom you are trying to seduce—nothing is more seductive to people than the feeling that they are desired.

Adventurousness. Charismatics are unconventional. They have an air of adventure and risk that attracts the bored. Be brazen and courageous in your actions—be seen taking risks for the good of others. Show heroism to give yourself a charisma that will last you a lifetime. Conversely, the slightest sign of cowardice or timidity will ruin whatever charisma you had.

Magnetism. If any physical attribute is crucial in seduction, it is the eyes. They reveal excitement, tension, detachment, without a word being spoken. The demeanor of Charismatics may be poised and calm, but their eyes are magnetic; they have a piercing gaze that disturbs their targets' emotions, exerting force without words or action. The eyes of the Charismatic never show fear or nerves.

Symbol: *The Lamp. Invisible to the eye, a current flowing through a wire in a glass vessel generates a heat that turns into candescence. All we see is the glow. In the prevailing darkness, the Lamp lights the way.*

the Star

Daily life is harsh, and most of us constantly seek escape from it in fantasies and dreams. Stars feed on this weakness; standing out from others through a distinctive and appealing style, they make us want to watch them. At the same time, they are vague and ethereal, keeping their distance, and letting us imagine more than is there. Their dreamlike quality works on our unconscious; we are not even aware how much we imitate them. Learn to become an object of fascination by projecting the glittering but elusive presence of the Star.

The cool, bright face which didn't ask for anything, which simply existed, waiting—it was an empty face, he thought; a face that could change with any wind of expression. One could dream into it anything. It was like a beautiful empty house waiting for carpets and pictures. It had all possibilities—it could become a palace or a brothel. It depended on the one who filled it. How limited by comparison was all that was already completed and labeled.

—ERICH MARIA REMARQUE, ON MARLENE DIETRICH, ARCH OF TRIUMPH

Keys to the Character

Seduction is a form of persuasion that seeks to bypass consciousness, stirring the unconscious mind instead. The reason for this is simple: we are so surrounded by stimuli that compete for our attention, bombarding us with obvious messages, and by people who are overtly political and manipulative, that we are rarely charmed or deceived by them. We have grown increasingly cynical. Try to persuade a person by appealing to their consciousness, by saying outright what you want, by showing all your cards, and what hope do you have? You are just one more irritation to be tuned out.

To avoid this fate you must learn the art of insinuation, of reaching the unconscious. The most eloquent expression of the unconscious is the dream, which is intricately connected to myth; waking from a dream, we are often haunted by its images and ambiguous messages. Dreams obsess us because they mix the real and the unreal. They are filled with real characters, and often deal with real situations, yet they are delightfully irrational, pushing realities to the extremes of delirium.

The gestures, the words, the very being of men like John F. Kennedy or Andy Warhol, for example, evoke both the real and the unreal: we may not realize it (and how could we, really), but they are like dream figures to us. They have qualities that anchor them in reality—sincerity, playfulness, sensuality—but at the same time their aloofness, their superiority, their almost surreal quality makes them seem like something out of a movie.

These types have a haunting, obsessive effect on people. Whether in public or in private, they seduce us, making us want to possess them both physically and psychologically. But how can we possess a person from a dream, or a movie star or political star, or even one of those real-life fascinators, like a Warhol, who may cross our path? Unable to have them, we become obsessed with them—they haunt our thoughts, our dreams, our fantasies. We imitate them unconsciously. That is the insidious seductive power of a Star, a power you can appropriate by making yourself into a cipher, a mix of the real and the unreal. Most people are hopelessly banal, that is, far too real. What you need to do is etherealize yourself. Your words and actions seem to come from your unconscious—have a certain looseness to them. You hold yourself back, occasionally revealing a trait that makes people wonder whether they really know you.

[John F.] Kennedy brought to television news and photojournalism the components most prevalent in the world of film: star quality and mythic story. With his telegenic looks, skills at self-presentation, heroic fantasies, and creative intelligence, Kennedy was brilliantly prepared to project a major screen persona. He appropriated the discourses of mass culture, especially of Hollywood, and transferred them to the news. By this strategy he made the news like dreams and like the movies— a realm in which images played out scenarios that accorded with the viewer's deepest yearnings ... Never appearing

The Star is a creation of modern cinema. And what enabled film to manufacture the Star was the close-up, which suddenly separates actors from their contexts, filling your mind with their image. Never forget this while fashioning yourself as a Star. First, you must have such a large presence that you can fill your target's mind the way a close-up fills the screen. You must have a style or presence that makes you stand out from everyone else. Be vague and dreamlike, yet not distant or absent—you don't want people to be unable to focus on or remember you. They have to be seeing you in their minds when you're not there.

Second, cultivate a blank, mysterious face, the center that radiates Starness. This allows people to read into you whatever they want to. Instead of signaling moods and emotions, instead of emoting or overemoting, the Star draws in interpretations.

A Star must stand out, and this may involve a certain dramatic flair. Sometimes, though, a more haunting, dreamlike effect can be created by subtle touches: the way you smoke a cigarette, a vocal inflection, a way of walking. It is often the little things that get under people's skin, and make them imitate you. Although these nuances may barely register to the conscious mind, subliminally they can be as attractive as an object with a striking shape or odd color. Unconsciously we are strangely drawn to things that have no meaning beyond their fascinating appearance.

Stars make us want to know more about them. You must learn to stir people's curiosity by letting them glimpse something in your private life—the causes you fight for, the person you are in love with (for the moment)—something that seems to reveal an element of your personality. Let them fantasize and imagine.

Another way Stars seduce is by making us identify with them, giving us a vicarious thrill. The key is to represent a type, as Jimmy Stewart represented the quintessential middle-American, Cary Grant the smooth aristocrat. People of your type will gravitate to you, identify with you, share your joy or pain. The attraction must be unconscious, conveyed not in your words but in your pose, your attitude.

You are an actor. And the most effective actors have an inner distance: they can mold their physical presence as if they perceived it from the outside. This inner distance fascinates us. Stars are playful about themselves, always adjusting their image, adapting it to the times. Nothing is more laughable than an image that was fashionable ten years ago but isn't any more. Stars must always

in an actual film, but rather turning the television apparatus into his screen, he became the greatest movie star of the twentieth century.

—JOHN HELLMANN, THE KENNEDY OBSESSION: THE AMERICAN MYTH OF JFK

> *The savage worships idols of wood and stone; the civilized man, idols of flesh and blood.*
> —George Bernard Shaw

renew their luster or face the worst possible fate: oblivion.

Symbol: *The Idol. A piece of stone carved into the shape of a god, perhaps glittering with gold and jewels. The eyes of the worshippers fill the stone with life, imagining it to have real powers. Its shape allows them to see what they want to see—a god—but it is actually just a piece of stone. The god lives in their imaginations.*

Part Two
the Seductive process

Most of us understand that certain actions on our part will have a pleasing and seductive effect on the person we would like to seduce. The problem is that we are generally too self-absorbed. We may occasionally do something that is seductive, but often we follow this up with a selfish or aggressive action (we are in a hurry to get what we want); or, unaware of what we are doing, we show a side of ourselves that is petty and banal, deflating any illusions or fantasies a person might have about us. Our attempts at seduction usually do not last long enough to create much of an effect.

You will not seduce anyone by simply depending on your engaging personality, or by occasionally doing something noble or alluring. Seduction is a process that occurs over time—the longer you take and the slower you go, the deeper you will penetrate into the mind of your victim.

The twenty-four chapters in this section will arm you with a series of tactics that will help you get out of yourself and into the mind of your victim, so that you can play it like an instrument.

The chapters are placed in a loose order, going from the initial contact with your victim to the successful conclusion. Because people's thoughts tend to revolve around their daily concerns and insecurities, you cannot proceed with a seduction until you slowly put their anxieties to sleep and fill their distracted minds with thoughts of you. The opening chapters will help you accomplish this. There is a natural tendency in relationships for people to become so familiar with one another that boredom and stagnation sets in. You have to constantly surprise your victims, stir things up, even shock them. The middle and later chapters will instruct you in the art of alternating hope and despair, pleasure and pain, until your victims weaken and succumb.

At all costs, resist the temptation to hurry to the climax of your seduction, or to improvise. You are not being seductive but selfish. Everything in daily life is hurried and improvised, and you need to offer something different. By taking your time and respecting the seductive process you will not only break down your victim's resistance, you will make them fall in love.

1
Choose the Right Victim

*Everything
depends on the target of your
seduction. Study your prey thoroughly, and choose only those who will
prove susceptible to your charms. The right victims are those for whom you can fill a void, who see
in you something exotic. They are often isolated or at
least somewhat unhappy (perhaps because of recent adverse circumstances), or can easily be made so—for the
completely contented person is almost impossible to seduce. The perfect victim has some natural quality that
attracts you. The strong emotions this quality inspires will help make your seductive maneuvers
seem more natural and dynamic. The perfect
victim allows for the perfect chase.*

Keys to Seduction

I have always noticed that men seldom fall in love with the most plastically beautiful women. There are a few "official beauties" in every society, whom people point to with their fingers in theaters and at parties, as if they were public monuments; however, personal masculine ardor is rarely directed toward them. Such beauty is so decidedly aesthetic that it converts the woman into an artistic object, and, by isolating her, places her at a distance ... The expressive charm of a certain manner of being, and not correctness or plastic perfection, is, in my opinion, the quality which effectively inspires love ... The idea of beauty, like a

Throughout life we find ourselves having to persuade people—to seduce them. Some will be relatively open to our influence, if only in subtle ways, while others seem impervious to our charms. Perhaps we find this a mystery beyond our control, but that is an ineffective way of dealing with life. Seducers prefer to pick the odds. As often as possible they go toward people who betray some vulnerability to them, and avoid the ones who cannot be moved. To leave people who are inaccessible to you alone is a wise path; you cannot seduce everyone. On the other hand, you must actively hunt out the prey that responds the right way.

How do you recognize your victims? By the way they respond to you. You should not pay so much attention to their conscious responses—a person who is obviously trying to please or charm you is probably playing to your vanity, and wants something from you. Instead, pay greater attention to those responses outside conscious control—a blush, an involuntary mirroring of some gesture of yours, an unusual shyness, even perhaps a flash of anger or resentment. All of these show that you are having an effect on a person who is open to your influence.

You can also recognize the right targets

by the effect they are having on you. Perhaps they make you uneasy—perhaps they correspond to a deep-rooted childhood ideal, or represent some kind of personal taboo that excites you. When a person has such a deep effect on you, it transforms all of your subsequent maneuvers. Your strong desire will infect the target and give them the dangerous sensation that they have a power over you.

Never rush into the waiting arms of the first person who seems to like you. That is not seduction but insecurity. The need that draws you will make for a low-level attachment, and interest on both sides will sag. Look at the types you have not considered before—that is where you will find challenge and adventure.

Although the victim who is perfect for you depends on you, certain types lend themselves to a more satisfying seduction. Just as it is hard to seduce a person who is happy, it is hard to seduce a person who has no imagination. People who are outwardly distant or shy are often better targets than extroverts. They are dying to be drawn out.

People with a lot of time on their hands are extremely susceptible to seduction. They have mental space for you to fill. On the other hand, you should generally avoid people who are preoccupied with business or work—seduction demands attention,

slab of magnificent marble, has crushed all possible refinement and vitality from the psychology of love.

—ORTEGA Y GASSET, *ON LOVE*, TRANSLATED BY TOBY TALBOT

> *It is a stroke of good fortune to find one who is worth seducing ... Most people rush ahead, become engaged or do other stupid things, and in a turn of the hand everything is over, and they know neither what they have won nor what they have lost.*
>
> —SÖREN KIERKEGAARD, *THE SEDUCER'S DIARY*

and busy people have too little space in their minds for you to occupy.

Your perfect victims are often people who think you have something they don't, and who will be enchanted to have it provided for them. Such victims may have a temperament quite the opposite of yours, and this difference will create an exciting tension.

Remember: the perfect victim is the person who stirs you in a way that cannot be explained in words. Be more creative in choosing your prey and you will be rewarded with a more exciting seduction.

> *For who so firm that cannot be seduced?*
>
> —WILLIAM SHAKESPEARE, *JULIUS CAESAR*

Symbol:

Big Game. Lions are dangerous—to hunt them is to know the thrill of risk. Leopards are clever and swift, offering the excitement of a difficult chase. Never rush into the hunt. Know your prey and choose it carefully. Do not waste time with small game—the rabbits that back into snares, the mink that walk into a scented trap. Challenge is pleasure.

2
Create a False Sense of Security—Approach Indirectly

If you are too direct early on, you risk stirring up a resistance that will never be lowered. At first there must be nothing of the seducer in your manner. The seduction should begin at an angle, indirectly, so that the target only gradually becomes aware of you. Haunt the periphery of your target's life—approach through a third party, or seem to cultivate a relatively neutral relationship, moving gradually from friend to lover. Arrange an occasional "chance" encounter, as if you and your target were destined to become acquainted—nothing is more seductive than a sense of destiny. Lull the target into feeling secure, then strike.

> *Many women adore the elusive, \ Hate overeagerness. So, play hard to get, \ Stop boredom developing. And don't let your entreaties \ Sound too confident of possession. Insinuate sex \ Camouflaged as friendship. I've seen ultrastubborn creatures \ Fooled by this gambit, the switch from companion to stud.*
>
> —OVID, THE ART OF LOVE, TRANSLATED BY PETER GREEN

Key to Seduction

What you are after as a seducer is the ability to move people in the direction you want them to go. But the game is perilous; the moment they suspect they are acting under your influence, they will become resentful. We are creatures who cannot stand feeling that we are obeying someone else's will. Should your targets catch on, sooner or later they will turn against you. But what if you can make them do what you want them to without their realizing it? What if they think *they* are in control? That is the power of indirection and no seducer can work his or her magic without it.

The first move to master is simple: once you have chosen the right person, you must make the target come to you. If, in the opening stages, you can make your targets think that they are the ones making the first approach, you have won the game. There will be no resentment, no perverse counterreaction, no paranoia.

To make them come to you requires giving them space. This can be accomplished in several ways. You can haunt the periphery of their existence, letting them notice you in different places but never approaching them. You will get their attention this way, and if they want to bridge the gap, they will have to come to you. You can play cat and mouse with them, first seeming interested, then stepping back—actively luring them to follow you into your web. Whatever you do, and whatever kind of seduction you are practicing, you must at all cost avoid the natural tendency to crowd your targets. Do not make the mistake of thinking they will lose interest unless you apply pressure, or that they will enjoy a flood of attention. Too much attention early on will actually just suggest insecurity, and raise doubts as to your motives. Worst of all, it gives your targets no room for imagination. Take a step back; let the thoughts you are provoking come to them as if they were their own.

In the initial stages of a seduction, you must find ways to calm any sense of mistrust that the other person may experience. (A sense of danger and fear can heighten the seduction later on, but if you stir such emotions in the first stages, you will more likely scare the target away.) Often the best way to seem harmless and to give yourself room to maneuver is to establish a friendship, moving steadily closer while always maintaining the distance appropriate for friends of the opposite sex. Your friendly conversations with your targets will bring you valuable information about their characters, their

> *On the street, I do not stop her, or I exchange a greeting with her but never come close, but always strive for distance. Presumably our repeated encounters are clearly noticeable to her; presumably she does perceive that on her horizon a new planet has loomed, which in its course has encroached disturbingly upon hers in a curiously undisturbing way, but she has no inkling of the law underlying this movement. ... Before I begin my attack, I must first become acquainted with her and her whole mental state.*
>
> —SØREN KIERKEGAARD, *THE SEDUCER'S DIARY*, TRANSLATED BY HOWARD V. HONG AND EDNA H. HONG

> *I had rather hear my dog bark at a crow than a man swear he loves me.*
>
> —BEATRICE, IN WILLIAM SHAKESPEARE, *MUCH ADO ABOUT NOTHING*

tastes, their weaknesses, the childhood yearnings that govern their adult behavior. In addition, by spending time with your targets you can make them comfortable with you. Believing you are interested only in their thoughts, in their company, they will lower their resistance, dissipating the usual tension between the sexes.

Now they are vulnerable, for your friendship with them has opened the golden gate to their body: their mind. At this point any offhand comment, any slight physical contact, will spark a different thought, which will catch them off-guard: perhaps there could be something else between you. Once that feeling has stirred, they will wonder why you haven't made a move, and will take the initiative themselves, enjoying the illusion that they are in control. There is nothing more effective in seduction than making the seduced think that they are the ones doing the seducing.

Symbol: The Spider's Web. The spider finds an innocuous corner in which to spin its web. The longer the web takes, the more fabulous its construction, yet few really notice it—its gossamer threads are nearly invisible. The spider has no need to chase for food, or even to move. It quietly sits in the corner, waiting for its victims to come to it on their own, and ensnare themselves in the web.

3
Send Mixed Signals

Once people are aware of your presence, and perhaps vaguely intrigued, you need to stir their interest before it settles on someone else. What is obvious and striking may attract their attention at first, but that attention is often short-lived; in the long run, ambiguity is much more potent. Most of us are much too obvious—instead, be hard to figure out. Send mixed signals: both tough and tender, both spiritual and earthy, both innocent and cunning. A mix of qualities suggests depth, which fascinates even as it confuses. An elusive, enigmatic aura will make people want to know more, drawing them into your circle. Create such a power by hinting at something contradictory within you.

Keys to Seduction

Nothing can proceed in seduction unless you can attract and hold your victim's attention, your physical presence becoming a haunting mental presence. It is actually quite easy to create that first stir—an alluring style of dress, a suggestive glance, something extreme about you. But what happens next? Our minds are barraged with images—not just from media but from the disorder of daily life. And many of these images are quite striking. You become just one more thing screaming for attention; your attractiveness will pass unless you spark the more enduring kind of spell that makes people think of you in your absence. That means engaging their imaginations, making them think there is more to you than what they see. Once they start embellishing your image with their fantasies, they are hooked.

This must, however, be done early on, before your targets know too much and their impressions of you are set. It should occur the moment they lay eyes on you. By sending mixed signals in that first encounter, you create a little surprise, a little tension: you seem to be one thing (innocent, brash, intellectual, witty), but you also throw them a glimpse of something else (devilish, shy, spontaneous, sad). Keep things subtle: if the second quality is

The idea that two distinct elements are combined in Mona Lisa's smile is one that has struck several critics. They accordingly find in the beautiful Florentine's expression the most perfect representation of the contrasts that dominate the erotic life of women; the contrast between reserve and seduction, and between the most devoted tenderness and a sensuality that is ruthlessly demanding—consuming men as if they were alien beings.

—SIGMUND FREUD, LEONARDO DA VINCI AND A MEMORY OF HIS CHILDHOOD, TRANSLATED BY ALAN TYSON

It is a universal truism that sexual attraction is enhanced by a certain amount of ambivalence. The true 100 per cent he-man is usually a little ridiculous rather than devastating. Japan, in particular, has a tradition of rather girlish heart-throbs. The jeune premier in romantic kabuki dramas is usually a pale, slim youth who invites maternal protection. The attraction of ambivalence appears to be as strong as ever. According to a recent poll in a woman's magazine the two "sexiest stars" of 1981 were Tamasaburo, a kabuki actor specializing in female roles, and Sawada Kenji, a pop singer who likes to perform

too strong, you will seem schizophrenic. But make them wonder why you might be shy or sad underneath your brash intellectual wit, and you will have their attention. Give them an ambiguity that lets them see what they want to see, capture their imagination with little voyeuristic glimpses into your dark soul.

To capture and hold attention, you need to show attributes that go against your physical appearance, creating depth and mystery. If you have a sweet face and an innocent air, let out hints of something dark, even vaguely cruel in your character. It is not advertised in your words, but in your manner. Do not worry if this underquality is a negative one, like danger, cruelty, or amorality; people will be drawn to the enigma anyway, and pure goodness is rarely seductive. Remember: no one is naturally mysterious, at least not for long; mystery is something you have to work at, a ploy on your part, and something that must be used early on in the seduction.

Playing with gender roles is a kind of intriguing paradox that has a long history in seduction. The greatest Don Juans have had a touch of prettiness and femininity, and the most attractive courtesans have had a masculine streak. The strategy, though, is only powerful when the underquality is merely hinted at; if the mix is too obvious or striking it will seem bizarre or even threatening.

A potent variation on this theme is the blending of physical heat and emotional coldness. Dandies like Beau Brummel and Andy Warhol combine striking physical appearances with a kind of coldness of manner, a distance from everything and everyone. They are both enticing and elusive, and people spend lifetimes chasing after such men, trying to shatter their unattainability. (The power of apparently unattainable people is devilishly seductive; we want to be the one to break them down.) They also wrap themselves in ambiguity and mystery, either talking very little or talking only of surface matters, hinting at a depth of character you can never reach.

Perhaps you have a reputation for a particular quality, which immediately comes to mind when people see you. You will better hold their attention by suggesting that behind this reputation some other quality lies lurking. No one had a darker, more sinful reputation than Lord Byron. What drove women wild was that behind his somewhat cold and disdainful exterior, they could sense that he was actually quite romantic, even spiritual. Byron played this up with his melancholic airs and occasional kind deed. Transfixed and confused, many women

in semidrag, more female than male.

—IAN BURUMA,
BEHIND THE MASK

thought that they could be the one to lead him back to goodness, to make him a faithful lover. Once a woman entertained such a thought, she was completely under his spell. It is not difficult to create such a seductive effect. Should you be known as eminently rational, say, hint at something irrational.

These principles have applications far beyond sexual seduction. To hold the attention of a broad public, to seduce them into thinking about you, you need to mix your signals. Display too much of one quality— even if it is a noble one, like knowledge or efficiency—and people will feel that you lack humanity. We are all complex and ambiguous, full of contradictory impulses; if you show only one side, even if it is your good side, you will wear on people's nerves. They will suspect you are a hypocrite. A bright surface may have a decorative charm, but what draws your eye into a painting is a depth of field, an inexpressible ambiguity, a surreal complexity.

Symbol:

The Theater Curtain. Onstage, the curtain's heavy deep-red folds attract your eye with their hypnotic surface. But what really fascinates and draws you in is what you think might be happening behind the curtain—the light peeking through, the suggestion of a secret, something about to happen. You feel the thrill of a voyeur about to watch a performance.

4
Appear to be an Object of Desire—Create Triangles

Few are drawn to the person whom others avoid or neglect; people gather around those who have already attracted interest. We want what other people want. To draw your victims closer and make them hungry to possess you, you must create an aura of desirability—of being wanted and courted by many. It will become a point of vanity for them to be the preferred object of your attention, to win you away from a crowd of admirers. Manufacture the illusion of popularity by surrounding yourself with members of the opposite sex— friends, former lovers, present suitors. Create triangles that stimulate rivalry and raise your value. Build a reputation that precedes you: if many have succumbed to your charms, there must be a reason.

Keys to Seduction

We are social creatures, and are immensely influenced by the tastes and desires of other people. Imagine a large social gathering. You see a man alone, whom nobody talks to for any length of time, and who is wandering around without company; isn't there a kind of self-fulfilling isolation about him? Why is he alone, why is he avoided? There has to be a reason. Until someone takes pity on this man and starts up a conversation with him, he will look unwanted and unwantable. But over there, in another corner, is a woman surrounded by people. They laugh at her remarks, and as they laugh, others join the group, attracted by its gaiety. When she moves around, people follow. Her face is glowing with attention. There has to be a reason.

In both cases, of course, there doesn't actually have to be a reason at all. The neglected man may have quite charming qualities, supposing you ever talk to him; but most likely you won't. Desirability is a social illusion. Its source is less what you say or do, or any kind of boasting or self-advertisement, than the sense that other people desire you. To turn your targets' interest into something deeper, into desire, you must make them see you as a person

Most of the time we prefer one thing to another because that is what our friends already prefer or because that object has marked social significance. Adults, when they are hungry, are just like children in that they seek out the foods that others take. In their love affairs, they seek out the man or woman whom others find attractive and abandon those who are not sought after. When we say of a man or woman that he or she is desirable, what we really mean is that others desire them. It is not that they have some particular quality, but because they conform to some currently modish model.

—SERGE MOSCOVICI, *THE AGE OF THE CROWD*, TRANS. J. C. WHITEHOUSE

It will be greatly to your advantage to entertain the lady you would win with an account of the number of women who are in love with you, and of the decided advances which they have made to you; for this will not only prove that you are a great favorite with the ladies, and a man of true honor, but it will convince her that she may have the honor of being enrolled in the same list, and of being praised in the same way, in the presence of your other female friends. This will greatly delight her.

—LOLA MONTEZ,
THE ARTS AND SECRETS OF BEAUTY, WITH HINTS TO GENTLEMEN ON THE ART OF FASCINATING

whom others cherish and covet. Make people compete for your attention, make them see you as sought after by everyone else. The aura of desirability will envelop you.

Your admirers can be friends or even suitors. Call it the harem effect. Pauline Bonaparte, sister of Napoleon, raised her value in men's eyes by always having a group of worshipful men around her at balls and parties. If she went for a walk, it was never with one man, always with two or three. Perhaps these men were simply friends, or even just props and hangers-on; the sight of them was enough to suggest that she was prized and desired, a woman worth fighting over. Andy Warhol, too, surrounded himself with the most glamorous, interesting people he could find. To be part of his inner circle meant that you were desirable as well. By placing himself in the middle but keeping himself aloof from it all, he made everyone compete for his attention. He stirred people's desire to possess him by holding back.

Practices like these not only stimulate competitive desires, they take aim at people's prime weakness: their vanity and self-esteem. We can endure feeling that another person has more talent, or more money, but the sense that a rival is more desirable than we are—that is unbearable. In the early eighteenth century, the Duke de Richelieu, a great rake, managed to seduce a young woman who was rather religious but whose husband, a dolt, was often away. He then proceeded to seduce her upstairs neighbor, a young widow. When the two women discovered that he was going from one to the other in the same night, they confronted him. A lesser man would have fled, but not the duke; he understood the dynamic of vanity and desire. Neither woman wanted to feel that he preferred the other. And so he managed to arrange a little ménage à trois, knowing that now they would struggle between themselves to be the favorite. When people's vanity is at risk, you can make them do whatever you want. According to Stendhal, if there is a woman you are interested in, pay attention to her sister. That will stir a triangular desire.

Your reputation—your illustrious past as a seducer—is an effective way of creating an aura of desirability. Women threw themselves at Errol Flynn's feet, not because of his handsome face, and certainly not because of his acting skills, but because of his reputation. They knew that other women had found him irresistible. Once he had established that reputation, he did not have to chase women anymore; they came to him. Your own reputation may not be so

> *It's annoying that our new acquaintance likes the boy. But aren't the best things in life free to all? The sun shines on everyone. The moon, accompanied by countless stars, leads even the beasts to pasture. What can you think of lovelier than water? But it flows for the whole world. Is love alone then something furtive rather than something to be gloried in? Exactly, that's just it—I don't want any of the good things of life unless people are envious of them.*
>
> —PETRONIUS, THE SATYRICON, TRANSLATED BY J. P. SULLIVAN

alluring, but you must find a way to suggest to your victim that others, many others, have found you desirable. It is reassuring. There is nothing like a restaurant-full of empty tables to persuade you not to go in.

A variation on the triangle strategy is the use of contrasts: careful exploitation of people who are dull or unattractive may enhance your desirability by comparison. At a social affair, for instance, make sure that your target has to chat with the most boring person available. Come to the rescue and your target will be delighted to see you. To make use of contrasts, either develop and display those attractive attributes (humor, vivacity, and so on) that are the scarcest in your own social group, or choose a group in which your natural qualities are rare, and will shine.

The use of contrasts has vast political ramifications, for a political figure must also seduce and seem desirable. Learn to play up the qualities that your rivals lack. In the American presidential race of 1980, the irresoluteness of Jimmy Carter made the single-mindedness of Ronald Reagan look desirable. Contrasts are eminently seductive because they do not depend on your own words or self-advertisements. The public reads them unconsciously, and sees what it wants to see.

Finally, appearing to be desired by others will raise your value, but often how you carry yourself can influence this as well. Do not let your targets see you so often; keep your distance, seem unattainable, out of their reach. An object that is rare and hard to obtain is generally more prized.

***Symbol:** The Trophy.*

What makes you want to win the trophy, and to see it as something worth having, is the sight of the other competitors. Some, out of a spirit of kindness, may want to reward everyone for trying, but the Trophy then loses its value. It must represent not only your victory but everyone else's defeat.

5
Create a Need—
Stir Anxiety and Discontent

A perfectly satisfied person cannot be seduced. Tension and disharmony must be instilled in your targets' minds. Stir within them feelings of discontent, an unhappiness with their circumstances and with themselves: their life lacks adventure, they have strayed from the ideals of their youth, they have become boring. The feelings of inadequacy that you create will give you space to insinuate yourself, to make them see you as the answer to their problems. Pain and anxiety are the proper precursors to pleasure. Learn to manufacture the need that you can fill.

Keys to Seduction

Everyone wears a mask in society; we pretend to be more sure of ourselves than we are. We do not want other people to glimpse that doubting self within us. In truth, our egos and personalities are much more fragile than they appear to be; they cover up feelings of confusion and emptiness. As a seducer, you must never mistake a person's appearance for the reality. People are always susceptible to being seduced, because in fact everyone lacks a sense of completeness, feels something missing deep inside. Bring their doubts and anxieties to the surface and they can be led and lured to follow you.

No one can see you as someone to follow or fall in love with unless they first reflect on themselves somehow, and on what they are missing. Before the seduction proceeds, you must place a mirror in front of them in which they glimpse that inner emptiness. Made aware of a lack, they now can focus on you as the person who can fill that empty space. Remember: most of us are lazy. To relieve our feelings of boredom or inadequacy on our own takes too much effort; letting someone else do the job is both easier and more exciting. The desire to have someone fill up our emptiness is the weakness on which all seducers prey. Make

We are all like pieces of the coins that children break in half for keepsakes—making two out of one, like the flatfish—and each of us is forever seeking the half that will tally with himself ... And so all this to-do is a relic of that original state of ours when we were whole, and now, when we are longing for and following after that primeval wholeness, we say we are in love.

—ARISTOPHANES'S SPEECH IN PLATO'S *SYMPOSIUM*, QUOTED IN JAMES MANDRELL, *DON JUAN AND THE POINT OF HONOR*

> *No one can fall in love if he is even partially satisfied with what he has or who he is. The experience of falling in love originates in an extreme depression, an inability to find something that has value in everyday life. The "symptom" of the predisposition to fall in love is not the conscious desire to do so, the intense desire to enrich our lives; it is the profound sense of being worthless and of having nothing that is valuable and the shame of not having it ... For this reason, falling in love occurs more frequently among young people, since they are profoundly uncertain, unsure of their worth, and often*

people anxious about the future, make them depressed, make them question their identity, make them sense the boredom that gnaws at their life. The ground is prepared. The seeds of seduction can be sown.

Your task as a seducer is to create a wound in your victim, aiming at their soft spot, the chink in their self-esteem. If they are stuck in a rut, make them feel it more deeply, "innocently" bringing it up and talking about it. What you want is an insecurity you can expand a little, an anxiety that can best be relieved by involvement with another person, namely you. They must feel the wound before they fall in love.

In your role of seducer, try to position yourself as coming from outside, as a stranger of sorts. You represent change, difference, a breakup of routines, the lure of the exotic. Make your victims feel that by comparison their lives are boring and their friends less interesting than they had thought. Remember: people prefer to feel that if their life is uninteresting, it is not because of themselves but because of their circumstances, the dull people they know, the town into which they were born. Once you make them feel the lure of the exotic, seduction is easy.

Another devilishly seductive area to aim at is the victim's past. To grow old is to renounce or compromise youthful ideals, to become less spontaneous, less alive in a way. This knowledge lies dormant in all of us. As a seducer you must bring it to the surface, make it clear how far people have strayed from their past goals and ideals. You, in turn, present yourself as representing that ideal, as offering a chance to recapture lost youth through adventure—through seduction. Old age is constantly seduced by youth, but first the young people must make it clear what the older ones are missing, how they have lost their ideals. Only then will they feel that the presence of the young will let them recapture that spark, the rebellious spirit that age and society have conspired to repress.

This concept has infinite applications. Corporations and politicians know that they cannot seduce their public into buying what they want them to buy, or doing what they want them to do, unless they first awaken a sense of need and discontent. Make the masses uncertain about their identity and you can help define it for them. It is as true of groups or nations as it is of individuals: they cannot be seduced without being made to feel some lack.

Part of John F. Kennedy's election strategy in 1960 was to make Americans unhappy about the 1950s, and how far the

ashamed of themselves. The same thing applies to people of other ages when they lose something in their lives—when their youth ends or when they start to grow old.

—Francesco Alberoni, *Falling in Love*, translated by Lawrence Venuti

Desire and love have for their object things or qualities which a man does not at present possess but which he lacks.

—Socrates, quoted in Plato's *Symposium*

The normal rhythm of life oscillates in general between a mild satisfaction with oneself and a slight discomfort, originating in the knowledge of one's personal shortcomings. We should like to be as handsome, young, strong or clever as other people of our acquaintance. We wish we could achieve as much as they do, long for similar advantages, positions, the same or greater success. To be delighted with oneself is the exception and, often enough, a smoke screen which we produce for ourselves and of course for others. Somewhere in it is a lingering feeling of discomfort with ourselves and a

country had strayed from its ideals. In talking about the '50s, he did not mention the nation's economic stability or its emergence as a superpower. Instead, he implied that the period was marked by conformity, a lack of risk and adventure, a loss of our frontier values. To vote for Kennedy was to embark on a collective adventure, to go back to ideals we had given up. But before anyone joined his crusade they had to be made aware of how much they had lost, what was missing. A group, like an individual, can get mired in routine, losing track of its original goals. Too much prosperity saps it of strength. You can seduce an entire nation by aiming at its collective insecurity, that latent sense that not everything is what it seems. Stirring dissatisfaction with the present and reminding people about the glorious past can unsettle their sense of identity. Then you can be the one to redefine it—a grand seduction.

Symbol: *Cupid's Arrow. What awakens desire in the seduced is not a soft touch or a pleasant sensation; it is a wound. The arrow creates a pain, an ache, a need for relief. Before desire there must be pain. Aim the arrow at the victim's weakest spot, creating a wound that you can open and reopen.*

slight self-dislike. I assert that an increase of this spirit of discontent renders a person especially susceptible to "falling in love." ... In most cases this attitude of disquiet is unconscious, but in some it reaches the threshold of awareness in the form of a slight uneasiness, or a stagnant dissatisfaction, or a realization of being upset without knowing why.

—Theodor Reik,
Of Love and Lust

6
Master the Art of Insinuation

Making your targets feel dissatisfied and in need of your attention is essential, but if you are too obvious, they will see through you and grow defensive. There is no known defense, however, against insinuation—the art of planting ideas in people's minds by dropping elusive hints that take root days later, even appearing to them as their own idea. Insinuation is the supreme means of influencing people. Create a sublanguage—bold statements followed by retraction and apology, ambiguous comments, banal talk combined with alluring glances—that enters the target's unconscious to convey your real meaning. Make everything suggestive.

Keys to Seduction

You cannot pass through life without in one way or another trying to persuade people of something. Take the direct route, saying exactly what you want, and your honesty may make you feel good but you are probably not getting anywhere. People have their own sets of ideas, which are hardened into stone by habit; your words, entering their minds, compete with the thousands of preconceived notions that are already there, and get nowhere. Besides, people resent your attempt to persuade them, as if they were incapable of deciding by themselves—as if you knew better. Consider instead the power of insinuation and suggestion. It requires some patience and art, but the results are more than worth it.

The way insinuation works is simple: disguised in a banal remark or encounter, a hint is dropped. It is about some emotional issue—a possible pleasure not yet attained, a lack of excitement in a person's life. The hint registers in the back of the target's mind, a subtle stab at his or her insecurities; its source is quickly forgotten. It is too subtle to be memorable at the time, and later, when it takes root and grows, it seems to have emerged naturally from the target's own mind, as if it was there all along. Insinuation lets you bypass people's natural resistance,

What distinguishes a suggestion from other kinds of psychical influence, such as a command or the giving of a piece of information or instruction, is that in the case of a suggestion an idea is aroused in another person's brain which is not examined in regard to its origin but is accepted just as though it had arisen spontaneously in that brain.

—SIGMUND FREUD

> *Glances are the heavy artillery of the flirt: everything can be conveyed in a look, yet that look can always be denied, for it cannot be quoted word for word.*
>
> —Stendhal, quoted in Richard Davenport-Hines, ed., *Vice: An Anthology*

for they seem to be listening only to what has originated in themselves. It is a language on its own, communicating directly with the unconscious. No seducer, no persuader, can hope to succeed without mastering the language and art of insinuation.

To sow a seductive idea you will need to engage people's imaginations, their fantasies, their deepest yearnings. What sets the wheels spinning is suggesting things that people want to hear—the possibility of pleasure, wealth, health, adventure. In the end, these good things turn out to be precisely what you seem to offer them. They will come to you as if on their own, unaware that you insinuated the idea in their heads.

Slips of the tongue, apparently inadvertent "sleep on it" comments, alluring references, statements for which you quickly apologize—all of these have immense insinuating power. They get under people's skin like a poison, and take on a life of their own. The key to succeeding with your insinuations is to make them when your targets are at their most relaxed or distracted, so that they are not aware of what is happening. Polite banter is often the perfect front for this; people are thinking about what they will say next, or are absorbed in their own thoughts. Your insinuations will barely register, which is how you want it.

In seduction, as the French courtesan Ninon de l'Enclos advised, it is better not to talk about your love for a person. Let your target read it in your manner. Your silence on the subject will have more insinuating power than if you had addressed it directly.

Not only words insinuate; pay attention to gestures and looks. Slight physical contact insinuates desire, as does an unusually warm tone of voice, both for the briefest of moments. The face speaks its own language. We are used to trying to read people's faces, which are often better indicators of their feelings than what they say, which is so easy to control. Since people are always reading your looks, use them to transmit the insinuating signals you choose—a fleeting but memorable glance, for instance.

Finally, the reason insinuation works so well is not just that it bypasses people's natural resistance. It is also the language of pleasure. There is too little mystery in the world; too many people say exactly what they feel or want. We yearn for something enigmatic, for something to feed our fantasies. Because of the lack of suggestion and ambiguity in daily life, the person who uses them suddenly seems to have something alluring and full of promise. It is a kind of titillating game—what is this person up to? Hints, suggestions, and insinuations create a seductive atmosphere, signaling that their victim is no longer involved in the routines of daily life but has entered another realm.

***Symbol:** The Seed.*
The soil is carefully prepared. The seeds are planted months in advance. Once they are in the ground, no one knows what hand threw them there. They are part of the earth. Disguise your manipulations by planting seeds that take root on their own.

7
Enter Their Spirit

*Most
people are locked in their
own worlds, making them stubborn
and hard to persuade. The way to lure them
out of their shell and set up your seduction is to
enter their spirit. Play by their rules, enjoy what they
enjoy, adapt yourself to their moods. In doing so you will
stroke their deep-rooted narcissism and lower their defenses.
Hypnotized by the mirror image you present, they will open up,
becoming vulnerable to your subtle influence. Soon you can
shift the dynamic: once you have entered their spirit you
can make them enter yours, at a point when it is
too late to turn back. Indulge your targets'
every mood and whim, giving them
nothing to react against or
resist.*

Keys to Seduction

One of the great sources of frustration in our lives is other people's stubbornness. How hard it is to reach them, to make them see things our way. We often have the impression that when they seem to be listening to us, and apparently agreeing with us, it is all superficial—the moment we are gone, they revert to their own ideas. We spend our lives butting up against people, as if they were stone walls. But instead of complaining about how misunderstood or ignored you are, why not try something different: instead of seeing other people as spiteful or indifferent, instead of trying to figure out why they act the way they do, look at them through the eyes of the seducer. The way to lure people out of their natural intractability and self-obsession is to enter their spirit.

All of us are narcissists. When we were children our narcissism was physical: we were interested in our own image, our own body, as if it were a separate being. As we grow older, our narcissism grows more psychological: we become absorbed in our own tastes, opinions, experiences. A hard shell forms around us. Paradoxically, the way to entice people out of this shell is to become more like them, in fact a kind of

You're anxious to keep your mistress? \ Convince her she's knocked you all of a heap \ With her stunning looks. If it's purple she's wearing, praise purple; \ When she's in a silk dress, say silk \ Suits her best of all ... Admire \ Her singing voice, her gestures as she dances, \ Cry "Encore!" when she stops. You can even praise \ Her performance in bed, her talent for love-making— \ Spell out what turned you on. \ Though she may show fiercer in action than any Medusa, \ Her lover will always describe her as kind \ And gentle. But take care not to give yourself away while \ Making such tongue-in-cheek compliments, mirror image of them. You do not have to spend days studying their minds; simply conform to their moods, adapt to their tastes, play along with whatever they send your way. In doing so you will lower their natural defensiveness. People truly love themselves, but what they love most of all is to see their ideas and tastes reflected in another person. This validates them. Their habitual insecurity vanishes. Hypnotized by their mirror image, they relax. Now you can slowly draw them out.

The difference between the sexes is what makes love and seduction possible, but it also involves an element of fear and distrust. A woman may fear male aggression and violence; a man is often unable to enter a woman's spirit, and so he remains strange and threatening. The greatest seducers in history grew up surrounded by women and had a touch of femininity themselves. The philosopher Sören Kierkegaard recommends spending more time with the opposite sex, getting to know the "enemy" and its weaknesses, so that you can turn this knowledge to your advantage.

Of all the seductive tactics, entering someone's spirit is perhaps the most devilish of all. It gives your victims the feeling that they are seducing you. The fact that you are indulging them, imitating them, entering

don't allow \Your expression to ruin the message. Art's most effective \ When concealed. Detection discredits you for good.

—OVID, *THE ART OF LOVE*, TRANSLATED BY PETER GREEN

Women are not at their ease except with those who take chances with them, and enter into their spirit.

—NINON DE L'ENCLOS

> *This desire for a double of the other sex that resembles us absolutely while still being other, for a magical creature who is ourself while possessing the advantage, over all our imaginings, of an autonomous existence ... We find traces of it in even the most banal circumstances of love ... The great, the implacable amorous passions are all linked to the fact that a being imagines he sees his most secret self spying upon him behind the curtain of another's eyes.*
>
> —Robert Musil, quoted in Denis de Rougemont, Love Declared, translated by Richard Howard

their spirit, suggests that you are under their spell. You are not a dangerous seducer to be wary of, but someone compliant and unthreatening. The attention you pay to them is intoxicating—since you are mirroring them, everything they see and hear from you reflects their own ego and tastes. What a boost to their vanity. All this sets up the seduction, the series of maneuvers that will turn the dynamic around. Once their defenses are down, they are open to your subtle influence. Soon you will begin to take over the dance, and without even noticing the shift, they will find themselves entering *your* spirit.

Symbol: *The Hunter's Mirror. The lark is a savory bird, but difficult to catch. In the field, the hunter places a mirror on a stand. The lark lands in front of the glass, steps back and forth, entranced by its own moving image and by the imitative mating dance it sees performed before its eyes. Hypnotized, the bird loses all sense of its surroundings, until the hunter's net traps it against the mirror.*

8
Create Temptation

Lure the target deep into your seduction by creating the proper temptation: a glimpse of the pleasures to come. As the serpent tempted Eve with the promise of forbidden knowledge, you must awaken a desire in your targets that they cannot control. Find that weakness of theirs, that fantasy that has yet to be realized, and hint that you can lead them toward it. It could be wealth, it could be adventure, it could be forbidden and guilty pleasures; the key is to keep it vague. Dangle the prize before their eyes, postponing satisfaction, and let their minds do the rest. The future seems ripe with possibility. Stimulate a curiosity stronger than the doubts and anxieties that go with it, and they will follow you.

Thou strong seducer, Opportunity.

—John Dryden

*Don Juan: Arminta, listen to the truth—for are not women friends of truth? I am a nobleman, heir to the ancient family of the Tenorios, the conquerors of Seville. After the king, my father is the most powerful and considered man at court ...
By chance I happened on this road and saw you. Love sometimes behaves in a manner that surprises even himself ...
• Arminta: I don't know if what you're saying is truth or lying rhetoric. I am married to Batricio, everybody knows it. How can the*

Keys to Seduction

Most of the time, people struggle to maintain security and a sense of balance in their lives. If they were always uprooting themselves in pursuit of every new person or fantasy that passed them by, they could not survive the daily grind. They usually win the struggle, but it does not come easy. The world is full of temptation. They read about people who have more than they do, about adventures others are having, about people who have found wealth and happiness. The security that they strive for, and that they seem to have in their lives, is actually an illusion. It covers up a constant tension.

As a seducer, you can never mistake people's appearance for reality. You know that their fight to keep order in their lives is exhausting, and that they are gnawed by doubts and regrets. It is hard to be good and virtuous, always having to repress the strongest desires. With that knowledge in mind, seduction is easier. What people want is not temptation; temptation happens every day. What people want is to give into temptation, to yield. That is the only way to get rid of the tension in their lives. It costs much more to resist temptation than to surrender.

Your task, then, is to create a temptation

that is stronger than the daily variety. It has to be focused on them, aimed at them as individuals—at their weakness. Understand: everyone has a principal weakness, from which others stem. Find that childhood insecurity, that lack in their life, and you hold the key to tempting them. Their weakness may be greed, vanity, boredom, some deeply repressed desire, a hunger for forbidden fruit. They signal it in little details that elude their conscious control: their style of clothing, an offhand comment. Their past, and particularly their past romances, will be littered with clues. Give them a potent temptation, tailored to their weakness, and you can make the hope of pleasure that you stir in them figure more prominently than the doubts and anxieties that accompany it.

A child has little power to resist. It wants everything, now, and rarely thinks of the consequences. A child lies lurking in everyone—a pleasure that was denied them, a desire that was repressed. Hit at that point, tempt them with the proper toy (adventure, money, fun), and they will slough off their normal adult reasonableness. Recognize their weakness by whatever childlike behavior they reveal in daily life—it is the tip of the iceberg.

Remember to keep the future gains vague, though, and somewhat out of reach.

marriage be annulled, even if he abandons me?
* *Don Juan: When the marriage is not consummated, whether by malice or deceit, it can be annulled ...*
* *Arminta: You are right. But, God help me, won't you desert me the moment you have separated me from my husband? ...*
* *Don Juan: Arminta, light of my eyes, tomorrow your beautiful feet will slip into polished silver slippers with buttons of the purest gold. And your alabaster throat will be imprisoned in beautiful necklaces; on your fingers, rings set with amethysts will shine like stars, and from your ears will dangle oriental*

> *pearls.*
> • *Arminta: I am yours.*
> —Tirso de Molina, The Playboy of Seville, translated by Adrienne M. Schizzano and Oscar Mandel, in Mandel, ed., The Theatre of Don Juan

Be too specific and you will disappoint; make the promise too close at hand, and you will not be able to postpone satisfaction long enough to get what you want.

Temptation is a twofold process. First you are coquettish, flirtatious; you stimulate a desire by promising pleasure and distraction from daily life. At the same time, you make it clear to your targets that they cannot have you, at least not right away. You are establishing a barrier, some kind of tension. The barriers and tensions in temptation are there to stop people from giving in too easily and too superficially. You *want* them to struggle, to resist, to be anxious.

In days gone by such barriers were easy to create, by taking advantage of preexisting social obstacles—of class, race, marriage, religion. Today the barriers have to be more psychological: your heart is taken by someone else; you are really not interested in the target; some secret holds you back; the timing is bad; you are not good enough for the other person; the other person is not good enough for you; and so on. Conversely, you can choose someone who has a built-in barrier: they are taken, they are not meant to want you.

These barriers are more subtle than the social or religious variety, but they are barriers nevertheless, and the psychology remains the same. People are perversely excited by what they cannot or should not have. Create this inner conflict—there is excitement and interest, but you are unavailable—and you will have them grasping for what they cannot reach. And the more your targets pursue you, the more they imagine that it is they who are aggressors. Your seduction is perfectly disguised.

Finally, the most potent temptations often involve psychological taboos and forbidden fruit. You are looking for some secret desire that will make your victim squirm uncomfortably if you hit upon it, but will tempt them all the more. Search in their past; whatever they seem to fear or flee from might hold the key. It could be a yearning for a mother or father figure, or a latent homosexual desire. Perhaps you can satisfy that desire by presenting yourself as a masculine woman or a feminine man. For others you play the Lolita, or the daddy—someone they are not supposed to have, the dark side of their personality. Then there are the masochists, the ones who secretly desire some pain. You can always tempt them by seeming difficult, challenging, even a little cruel. Keep the connection vague—you want them to grab at something elusive, something that comes out of their own mind.

The only way to get rid of temptation is to yield to it.

—OSCAR WILDE

Symbol:
The Apple in the Garden of Eden. The fruit looks deeply inviting, and you are not supposed to eat of it; it is forbidden. But that is precisely why you think of it day and night. You see it but cannot have it. And the only way to get rid of this temptation is to yield and taste the fruit.

9
Keep Them in Suspense—
What Comes Next?

The moment people feel they know what to expect from you, your spell on them is broken. More: you have ceded them power. The only way to lead the seduced along and keep the upper hand is to create suspense, a calculated surprise. People love a mystery, and this is the key to luring them further into your web. Behave in a way that leaves them wondering, What are you up to? Doing something they do not expect from you will give them a delightful sense of spontaneity—they will not be able to foresee what comes next. You are always one step ahead and in control. Give the victim a thrill with a sudden change of direction.

> *I count upon taking [the French people] by surprise. A bold deed upsets people's equanimity, and they are dumbfounded by a great novelty.*
>
> —NAPOLEON BONAPARTE, QUOTED IN EMIL LUDWIG, *NAPOLEON*, TRANSLATED BY EDEN AND CEDAR PAUL

Keys to Seduction

A child is usually a willful, stubborn creature who will deliberately do the opposite of what we ask. But there is one scenario in which children will happily give up their usual willfulness: when they are promised a surprise. Perhaps it is a present hidden in a box, a game with an unforeseeable ending, a journey with an unknown destination, a suspenseful story with a surprise finish. In those moments when children are waiting for a surprise, their willpower is suspended. They are in your thrall for as long as you dangle possibility before them. This childish habit is buried deep within us, and is the source of an elemental human pleasure: being led by a person who knows where they are going, and who takes us on a journey. (Maybe our joy in being carried along involves a buried memory of being literally carried, by a parent, when we are small.)

We get a similar thrill when we watch a movie or read a thriller: we are in the hands of a director or author who is leading us along, taking us through twists and turns. We stay in our seats, we turn the pages, happily enslaved by the suspense. It is the pleasure a woman has in being led by a confident dancer, letting go of any defensiveness she may feel and letting another person do the work. Falling in love involves anticipation; we are about to head off in a new direction, enter a new life, where everything will be strange. The seduced wants to be led, to be carried along like a child. If you are predictable, the charm wears off; everyday life is predictable. Your targets must never know what's coming next—what surprises you have in store for them. As with a child, their natural willfulness will be suspended for as long as you can keep them guessing.

There are all kinds of calculated surprises you can spring on your victims—sending a letter from out of the blue, taking them to a place they have never been. But best of all are surprises that reveal something new about your character. This needs to be set up. In those first few weeks, your targets will tend to make certain snap judgments about you, based on appearances. Perhaps they see you as a bit shy, practical, puritanical. You know that this is not the real you, but it is how you act in social situations. Let them, however, have these impressions, and in fact accentuate them a little, without overacting: for instance, seem a little more reserved than usual. Now you have room to suddenly surprise them with some bold or poetic or naughty action. Once they have changed their minds about

> *This is always the law for the interesting ...: If one just knows how to surprise, one always wins the game. The energy of the person involved is temporarily suspended; one makes it impossible for her to act.*
>
> —SÖREN KIERKEGAARD, *THE SEDUCER'S DIARY*

you, surprise them again. As they strain to figure you out, they will be thinking about you all of the time.

Surprise creates a moment when people's defenses come down and new emotions can rush in. If the surprise is pleasurable, the seductive poison enters their veins without them realizing it. Any sudden event has a similar effect, striking directly at our emotions before we get defensive.

Not only does suddenness create a seductive jolt, it conceals manipulations. Appear somewhere unexpectedly, say or do something sudden, and people will not have time to figure out that your move was calculated. Take them to some new place as if it only just occurred to you, suddenly reveal some secret. Made emotionally vulnerable, they will be too bewildered to see through you. Anything that happens suddenly seems natural, and anything that seems natural has a seductive charm.

If you are in the public eye, you must learn from this trick of surprise. People are bored, not only with their own lives but with people who are meant to keep them from being bored. The minute they feel they can predict your next step, they will eat you alive. The artist Andy Warhol kept moving from incarnation to incarnation, and no one could predict the next one—artist, filmmaker, society man. Always keep a surprise up your sleeve. To keep the public's attention, keep them guessing. Let the moralists accuse you of insincerity, of having no core or center. They are actually jealous of the freedom and playfulness you reveal in your public persona.

***Symbol:** The Roller Coaster. The car rises slowly to the top, then suddenly hurtles you into space, whips you to the side, throws you upside down, in every possible direction. The riders laugh and scream. What thrills them is to let go, to grant control to someone else, who propels them in unexpected directions. What new thrill awaits them around the next corner?*

10
Use the Demonic Power of Words to Sow Confusion

*It
is hard to make
people listen; they are consumed
with their own thoughts and desires, and
have little time for yours. The trick to making them
listen is to say what they want to hear, to fill their ears
with whatever is pleasant to them. This is the essence of seductive language. Inflame people's emotions with loaded phrases,
flatter them, comfort their insecurities, envelop them in fantasies,
sweet words, and promises, and not only will they listen to you,
they will lose their will to resist you. Keep your language
vague, letting them read into it what they
want. Use writing to stir up fantasies
and to create an idealized
portrait of your-
self.*

Keys to Seduction

We rarely think before we talk. It is human nature to say the first thing that comes into our head—and usually what comes first is something about ourselves. We primarily use words to express our own feelings, ideas, and opinions. (Also to complain and to argue.) This is because we are generally self-absorbed—the person who interests us most is our own self. To a certain extent this is inevitable, and through much of our lives there is nothing much wrong with it; we can function quite well this way. In seduction, however, it limits our potential.

You cannot seduce without an ability to get outside your own skin and inside another person's, piercing their psychology. The key to seductive language is not the words you utter, or your seductive tone of voice; it is a radical shift in perspective and habit. You have to stop saying the first thing that comes to your mind—you have to control the urge to prattle and vent your opinions. The key is to see words as a tool not for communicating true thoughts and feelings but for confusing, delighting, and intoxicating.

The difference between normal language and seductive language is like the difference between noise and music. Noise is a

Therefore, the person who is unable to write letters and notes never becomes a dangerous seducer.

—SØREN KIERKEGAARD, EITHER/OR, TRANSLATED BY HOWARD V. HONG AND EDNA H. HONG

That man that hath a tongue, I say, is no man, / If with his tongue he cannot win a woman.

—WILLIAM SHAKESPEARE, THE TWO GENTLEMEN OF VERONA

My mistress staged a lock-out ... \ I went back to verses and compliments, \ My natural weapons. Soft words \ Remove harsh door-chains. There's magic in poetry, its power \ Can pull down the bloody moon, \ Turn back the sun, make serpents burst asunder \ Or rivers flow upstream. \ Doors are no match for such spellbinding, the toughest \ Locks can be open-sesamed by its charms. \ But epic's a dead loss for me. I'll get nowhere with swift-footed \ Achilles, or with either of Atreus' sons. \ Old what's-his-name wasting twenty years on war and travel, \ Poor Hector dragged in the dust— \ No good. But lavish

constant in modern life, something irritating we tune out if we can. Our normal language is like noise—people may half-listen to us as we go on about ourselves, but just as often their thoughts are a million miles away. Every now and then their ears prick up when something we say touches on them, but this lasts only until we return to yet another story about ourselves. As early as childhood we learn to tune out this kind of noise (particularly when it comes from our parents).

Music, on the other hand, is seductive, and gets under our skin. It is intended for pleasure. A melody or rhythm stays in our blood for days after we have heard it, altering our moods and emotions, relaxing or exciting us. To make music instead of noise, you must say things that please—things that relate to people's lives, that touch their vanity. If they have many problems, you can produce the same effect by distracting them, focusing their attention away from themselves by saying things that are witty and entertaining, or that make the future seem bright and hopeful. Promises and flattery are music to anyone's ears. These are words designed to move people and lower their resistance.

Flattery is seductive language in its purest form. Its purpose is not to express a truth or a real feeling, but only to create an effect on the recipient. Learn to sniff out the parts of a person's ego that need validation and then aim your flattery directly at such insecurities. Make it a surprise, something no one else has thought to flatter before—something you can describe as a talent or positive quality that others had not noticed.

The most anti-seductive form of language is argument. How many silent enemies do we create by arguing? There is a superior way to get people to listen and be persuaded: humor and a light touch. Laughter and applause have a domino effect: once your listeners have laughed, they are more likely to laugh again. In this lighthearted mood they are also more apt to listen. A subtle touch and a bit of irony give you room to persuade them, move them to your side, mock your enemies. That is the seductive form of argument.

If speaking before a group, your seductive language should aim at your audience's emotions, for emotional people are easier to deceive. Everyone shares emotions, and no one feels inferior to a speaker who stirs up their feelings. The crowd bonds together, everyone contagiously experiencing the same passionate sentiments. The emotions you are trying to arouse should be strong ones. Do not speak of friendship and dis-

fine words on some young girl's profile \ And sooner or later she'll tender herself as the fee, \ An ample reward for your labors. So farewell, heroic \ Figures of legend—the quid \ Pro quo you offer won't tempt me. A bevy of beauties \ All swooning over my love-songs— that's what I want.

—OVID, THE AMORES, TRANSLATED BY PETER GREEN

agreement; speak of love and hate. And it is crucial to try to feel something of the emotions you are trying to elicit. You will be more believable that way.

The goal of seductive speech is often to create a kind of hypnosis: you are distracting people, lowering their defenses, making them more vulnerable to suggestion. Learn the hypnotist's lessons of repetition and affirmation, key elements in putting a subject to sleep. Affirmation is simply the making of strong positive statements, like the hypnotist's commands. Seductive language should have a kind of boldness, which will cover up a multitude of sins. Your audience will be so caught up in your bold language that they won't have time to reflect on whether or not it is true. Never say, "I don't think the other side made a wise decision"; say "We deserve better," or "They have made a mess of things." Affirmative language is active language, full of verbs, imperatives, and short sentences. Cut out "I believe," "Perhaps," "In my opinion." Head straight for the heart.

Learn to incorporate seductive language into your writing, particularly in any letters to your target. With an intimate letter, you are in complete control of the dynamic, able to move your victims' emotions in the proper direction, infect them with desire. It is best not to begin your correspondence until at least several weeks after your initial contact. Let your victims get an impression of you: you seem intriguing, yet you show no particular interest in them. When you sense that they are thinking about you, that is the time to hit them with your first letter. Any desire you express for them will come as a surprise; their vanity will be tickled and they will want more.

Design your letters as homages to your targets. Make everything you write come back to them, as if they were all you could think about—a delirious effect. If you tell an anecdote, make it somehow relate to them. Your correspondence is a kind of mirror you are holding up to them—they get to see themselves reflected through your desire.

A letter can suggest emotion by seeming disordered, rambling from one subject to another. Clearly it is hard for you to think; your love has unhinged you. Disordered thoughts are exciting thoughts. Do not waste time on real information; focus on feelings and sensations, using expressions that are ripe with connotation. Do not become sentimental—it is tiring, and too direct. Better to suggest the effect your target has on you than to gush about how you feel. Stay vague and ambiguous, allowing the reader the space to imagine and fantasize. The goal of your writing is not to express yourself but to create emotion in the reader, spreading confusion and desire.

You will know that your letters are having the proper effect when your targets come to mirror your thoughts, repeating words you wrote, whether in their own letters or in person. This is the time to move to the more physical and erotic. Use language that quivers with sexual connotation, or, better still, suggest sexuality by making your letters shorter, more frequent, and even more disordered than before. There is nothing more erotic than the short abrupt note. Your thoughts are unfinished; they can only be completed by the other person.

Symbol: *The Clouds. In the clouds it is hard to see the exact forms of things. Everything seems vague; the imagination runs wild, seeing things that are not there. Your words must lift people into the clouds, where it is easy for them to lose their way.*

11
Pay Attention to Detail

Lofty words and grand gestures can be suspicious: why are you trying so hard to please? The details of a seduction—the subtle gestures, the offhand things you do—are often more charming and revealing. You must learn to distract your victims with a myriad of pleasant little rituals—thoughtful gifts tailored just for them, clothes and adornments designed to please them, gestures that show the time and attention you are paying them. All of their senses are engaged in the details you orchestrate. Create spectacles to dazzle their eyes; mesmerized by what they see, they will not notice what you are really up to. Learn to suggest the proper feelings and moods through details.

> *Therefore in my view when the courtier wishes to declare his love he should do so by his actions rather than by speech, for a man's feelings are sometimes more clearly revealed by ... a gesture of respect or a certain shyness than by volumes of words.*
>
> — BALDASSARE CASTIGLIONE, THE BOOK OF THE COURTIER

Keys to Seduction

When we were children, our senses were much more active. The colors of a new toy, or a spectacle such as a circus, held us in thrall; a smell or a sound could fascinate us. In the games we created, many of them reproducing something in the adult world on a smaller scale, what pleasure we took in orchestrating every detail. We noticed everything.

As we grow older our senses get dulled. We no longer notice as much, for we are constantly hurrying to get things done, to move on to the next task. In seduction, you are always trying to bring the target back to the golden moments of childhood. A child is less rational, more easily deceived. A child is also more attuned to the pleasures of the senses. So when your targets are with you, you must never give them the feeling they normally get in the real world, where we are all rushed, ruthless, out for ourselves. You need to deliberately slow things down, and return them to the simpler times of their youth. The details that you orchestrate—colors, gifts, little ceremonies—are aimed at their senses, at the childish delight we take in the immediate charms of the natural world. Their senses filled with delightful things, they grow less capable of reason and rationality. Pay attention to detail and you will find yourself assuming a slower pace; your targets will not focus on what you might be after (sexual favors, power, etc.) because you seem so considerate, so attentive. In the childish realm of the senses in which you envelop them, they get a clear sense that you are involving them in something distinct from the real world—an essential ingredient of seduction.

From the 1940s on into the early 1960s, Pamela Churchill Harriman had a series of affairs with some of the most prominent and wealthy men in the world. What attracted these men, and kept them in thrall, was not her beauty or her lineage or her vivacious personality, but her extraordinary attention to detail. It began with her attentive look as she listened to your every word, soaking up your tastes. Once she found her way into your home, she would fill it with your favorite flowers, get your chef to cook that dish you had only tasted in the finest restaurants. You mentioned an artist you liked? A few days later that artist would be attending one of your parties. She found the perfect antiques for you, dressed in the way that most pleased or excited you, and she did this without your saying a word—she spied, gathered information from third parties, overheard you talking to someone else. Harriman's attention to detail had an intoxicating effect on all the men in her life. Life is harsh and competitive. Attending to detail in a way that is soothing to the other person makes them dependent upon you. The key is probing their needs in a way that is not too obvious, so that when you make precisely the right gesture, it seems uncanny, as if you had read their mind.

Everything in seduction is a sign, and none more so than clothes. It is not that you have to dress interestingly, elegantly, or provocatively, but that you have to dress for your target—have to appeal to your target's tastes. When Cleopatra was seducing Mark Antony, her dress was not brazenly sexual; she dressed as a Greek goddess, knowing his weakness for such fantasy figures. Madame de Pompadour, the mistress of King Louis XV, knew the king's weakness, his chronic boredom; she constantly wore different clothes, changing not only their color but their style, supplying the King with a constant feast for his eyes. Contrast works well here: at work or at home, you might dress nonchalantly, but when you are with the target you wear something elaborate, as if you were putting on a costume. Your Cinderella transformation will stir excitement, and the feeling that you have done something just for the person you are with.

A gift has immense seductive power, but the object itself is less important than the gesture, and the subtle thought or emotion that it communicates. Perhaps the choice relates to something from the target's past, or symbolizes something between you, or merely represents the lengths you will go to to please. Expensive gifts have no sentiment attached; they may temporarily excite their recipient but they are quickly forgotten, as a child forgets a new toy. The object that reflects its giver's attentiveness has a lingering sentimental power, which resurfaces every time its owner sees it.

Finally, words are important in seduction, and have a great deal of power to confuse, distract, and boost the vanity of the target. But what is most seductive in the long run is what you do not say, what you communicate indirectly. Words come easily, and people distrust them. Anyone can say the right words; and once they are said, nothing is binding, and they may even be forgotten altogether. The gesture, the thoughtful gift, the little details seem much more real and substantial. They are also much more charming than lofty words about love, precisely because they speak for themselves and let the seduced read into them more than is there. Never tell someone what you are feeling; let them guess it in your looks and gestures. That is the more convincing language.

Symbol:

The Banquet. A feast has been prepared in your honor. Everything has been elaborately coordinated—the flowers, the decorations, the selection of guests, the dancers, the music, the five-course meal, the endlessly flowing wine. The Banquet loosens your tongue, and also your inhibitions.

12
Poeticize Your Presence

*Important things happen
when your targets are alone: the
slightest feeling of relief that you are not
there, and it is all over. Familiarity and overexposure will cause this reaction. Remain elusive,
then, so that when you are away, they will yearn to
see you again, and will associate you only with pleasant
thoughts. Occupy their minds by alternating an exciting
presence with a cool distance, exuberant moments followed by calculated absences. Associate yourself with poetic images and objects, so that when they think of you,
they begin to see you through an idealized halo. The
more you figure in their minds, the more they will
envelop you in seductive fantasies. Feed these
fantasies by subtle inconsistencies and
changes in your behavior.*

> *He who does not know how to encircle a girl so that she loses sight of everything he does not want her to see, he who does not know how to poetize himself into a girl so that it is from her that everything proceeds as he wants it—he is and remains a bungler ... To poetize oneself into a girl is an art.*
>
> —Søren Kierkegaard, *The Seducer's Diary*, translated by Howard V. Hong and Edna H. Hong

Keys to Seduction

We all have a self-image that is more flattering than the truth: we think of ourselves as more generous, selfless, honest, kindly, intelligent, or good-looking than in fact we are. It is extremely difficult for us to be honest with ourselves about our own limitations; we have a desperate need to idealize ourselves. As the writer Angela Carter remarks, we would rather align ourselves with angels than with the higher primates from which we are actually descended.

This need to idealize extends to our romantic entanglements, because when we fall in love, or under the spell of another person, we see a reflection of ourselves. The choice we make in deciding to become involved with another person reveals something important and intimate about us: we resist seeing ourselves as having fallen for someone who is cheap or tacky or tasteless, because it reflects badly on who we are. Furthermore, we are often likely to fall for someone who resembles us in some way. Should that person be deficient, or worst of all ordinary, then there is something deficient and ordinary about us. No, at all costs the loved one must be overvalued and idealized, at least for the sake of our own self-esteem. Besides, in a world that is harsh and full of disappointment, it is a great pleasure to be able to fantasize about a person you are involved with.

This makes the seducer's task easy: people are dying to be given the chance to fantasize about *you*. Do not spoil this golden opportunity by overexposing yourself, or becoming so familiar and banal that the target sees you exactly as you are. You do not have to be an angel, or a paragon of virtue—that would be quite boring. You can be dangerous, naughty, even somewhat vulgar, depending on the tastes of your victim. But never be ordinary or limited. In poetry (as opposed to reality), anything is possible.

To make your targets idealize you it is critical that you add an element of doubt—you might not be that interested in them, you are somewhat elusive. Remember: if you are easily had, you cannot be worth that much. It is hard to wax poetic about a person who comes so cheaply. If, after the initial interest, you make it clear that you cannot be taken for granted, if you stir a bit of doubt, the target will imagine there is something special, lofty, and unattainable about you.

People get deep pleasure from associating others with some kind of childhood fantasy figure. John F. Kennedy presented himself as a figure out of chivalry. Pablo

> *What I need is a woman who is something, anything; either very beautiful or very kind or in the last resort very wicked; very witty or very stupid, but something.*
>
> —ALFRED DE MUSSET

Picasso was not just a great painter with a thirst for young girls, he was the Minotaur of Greek legend, or the devilish trickster figure that is so seductive to women. These associations should not be made too early; they are only powerful once the target has begun to fall under your spell. The trick is to associate your image with something mythic and poetic, through the clothes you wear, the things you say, the places you go.

Any kind of heightened experience, artistic or spiritual, lingers in the mind much longer than normal experience. You must find a way to share such moments with your targets—a concert, a play, a spiritual encounter, whatever it takes—so that they associate something elevated with you. Shared moments of exuberance have immense seductive pull. Also, any kind of object can be imbued with poetic resonance and sentimental associations, as discussed in the last chapter. The gifts you give and other objects can become imbued with your presence; if they are associated with pleasant memories, the sight of them keeps you in mind and accelerates the poeticization process.

Although it is said that absence makes the heart grow fonder, an absence too early will prove deadly. You must surround your targets with focused attention, so that in those critical moments when they are alone, their mind is spinning with a kind of afterglow. Do everything you can to keep the target thinking about you. Letters, mementos, gifts, unexpected meetings—all these give you a poetic omnipresence. Everything must remind them of you.

Symbol: *The Halo.*

Slowly, when the target is alone, he or she begins to imagine a kind of faint glow around your head, formed by all of the possible pleasures you might offer, the radiance of your charged presence, your noble qualities. The Halo separates you from other people. Do not make it disappear by becoming familiar and ordinary.

13
Disarm Through Strategic Weakness and Vulnerability

Too much maneuvering on your part may raise suspicion. The best way to cover your tracks is to make the other person feel superior and stronger. If you seem to be weak, vulnerable, enthralled by the other person, and unable to control yourself, you will make your actions look more natural, less calculated. Physical weakness—tears, bashfulness, paleness—will help create the effect. To further win trust, exchange honesty for virtue: establish your "sincerity" by confessing some sin on your part—it doesn't have to be real. Sincerity is more important than goodness. Play the victim, then transform your target's sympathy into love.

Keys to Seduction

We all have weaknesses, vulnerabilities, frailnesses in our mental makeup. Perhaps we are shy or oversensitive, or need attention—whatever the weakness is, it is something we cannot control. We may try to compensate for it, or to hide it, but this is often a mistake: people sense something inauthentic or unnatural. Remember: what is natural to your character is inherently seductive. A person's vulnerability, what they seem to be unable to control, is often what is most seductive about them. People who display no weaknesses, on the other hand, often elicit envy, fear, and anger—we want to sabotage them just to bring them down.

Do not struggle against your vulnerabilities, or try to repress them, but put them into play. Learn to transform them into power. The game is subtle: if you wallow in your weakness, overplay your hand, you will be seen as angling for sympathy, or, worse, as pathetic. No, what works best is to allow people an occasional glimpse into the soft, frail side of your character, and usually only after they have known you for a while. That glimpse will humanize you, lowering their suspicions, and preparing the ground for a deeper attachment. Normally strong and in control, at moments you let go, give in to your weakness, let them see it.

Ordinarily, young girls speak very harshly about bashful men, but secretly they like them. A little bashfulness flatters a teenage girl's vanity, makes her feel superior; it is her earnest money. When they are lulled to sleep, then at the very time they believe you are about to perish from bashfulness, you show them that you are so far from it that you are quite self-reliant. Bashfulness makes a man lose his masculine significance, and therefore it is a relatively good means for neutralizing the sex relation.

—SØREN KIERKEGAARD, THE SEDUCER'S DIARY, TRANSLATED BY HOWARD AND EDNA HONG

> *The weak ones do have a power over us. The clear, forceful ones I can do without. I am weak and indecisive by nature myself, and a woman who is quiet and withdrawn and follows the wishes of a man even to the point of letting herself be used has much the greater appeal. A man can shape and mold her as he wishes, and becomes fonder of her all the while.*
>
> —Murasaki Shikibu, The Tale of Genji, translated by Edward G. Seidensticker

There are fears and insecurities peculiar to each sex; your use of strategic weakness must always take these differences into account. A woman, for instance, may be attracted by a man's strength and self-confidence, but too much of it can create fear, seeming unnatural, even ugly. Particularly intimidating is the sense that the man is cold and unfeeling. She may feel insecure that he is only after sex, and nothing else. Male seducers long ago learned to become more feminine—to show their emotions, and to seem interested in their targets' lives.

Some of the greatest seducers in recent history—Gabriele d'Annunzio, Duke Ellington, Errol Flynn—understood the value of acting slavishly to a woman, like a troubadour on bended knee. The key is to indulge your softer side while still remaining as masculine as possible. This may include an occasional show of bashfulness, which the philosopher Sören Kierkegaard thought an extremely seductive tactic for a man—it gives the woman a sense of comfort, and even of superiority. Remember, though, to keep everything in moderation. A glimpse of shyness is sufficient; too much of it and the target will despair, afraid that she will end up having to do all the work.

A man's fears and insecurities often concern his sense of masculinity; he usually will feel threatened by a woman who is too overtly manipulative, who is too much in control. The greatest seductresses in history knew how to cover up their manipulations by playing the little girl in need of masculine protection. To make this most effective, a woman should seem both in need of protection and sexually excitable, giving the man his ultimate fantasy.

Seeing someone cry usually has an immediate effect on our emotions: we cannot remain neutral. We feel sympathy, and most often will do anything to stop the tears—including things that we normally would not do. Weeping is an incredibly potent tactic, but the weeper is not always so innocent. There is usually something real behind the tears, but there may also be an element of acting, of playing for effect. (And if the target senses this the tactic is doomed.) Beyond the emotional impact of tears, there is something seductive about sadness. We want to comfort the other person, and that desire quickly turns into love.

Use tears sparingly, and save them for the right moment. Perhaps this might be a time when the target seems suspicious of your motives, or when you are worrying about having no effect on him or her. Tears are a sure barometer of how deeply the other person is falling for you. If they seem

You know, a man ain't worth a damn if he can't cry at the right time.

—Lyndon Baines Johnson

annoyed, or resist the bait, your case is probably hopeless.

In social and political situations, seeming too ambitious, or too controlled, will make people fear you; it is crucial to show your soft side. The display of a single weakness will hide a multitude of manipulations. Emotion or even tears will work here too. Most seductive of all is playing the victim. Attacking your mean-spirited opponents can make you seem ugly as well; instead, soak up their blows, and play the victim. The public will rally to your side, in an emotional response that will lay the groundwork for a grand political seduction.

Symbol: The Blemish. A beautiful face is a delight to look at, but if it is too perfect it leaves us cold, and even slightly intimidated. It is the little mole, the beauty mark, that makes the face human and lovable. So do not conceal all of your blemishes. You need them to soften your features and elicit tender feelings.

14
Confuse Desire and Reality— The Perfect Illusion

To compensate for the difficulties in their lives, people spend a lot of their time daydreaming, imagining a future full of adventure, success, and romance. If you can create the illusion that through you they can live out their dreams, you will have them at your mercy. It is important to start slowly, gaining their trust, and gradually constructing the fantasy that matches their desires. Aim at secret wishes that have been thwarted or repressed, stirring up uncontrollable emotions, clouding their powers of reason. The perfect illusion is one that does not depart too much from reality, but has a touch of the unreal to it, like a waking dream. Lead the seduced to a point of confusion in which they can no longer tell the difference between illusion and reality.

> *Lovers and madmen have such seething brains, \ Such shaping fantasies, that apprehend \ More than cool reason ever comprehends.*
>
> —WILLIAM SHAKESPEARE, A MIDSUMMER NIGHT'S DREAM

Keys to Seduction

The real world can be unforgiving: events occur over which we have little control, other people ignore our feelings in their quests to get what they need, time runs out before we accomplish what we had wanted. If we ever stopped to look at the present and future in a completely objective way, we would despair. Fortunately we develop the habit of dreaming early on. In this other, mental world that we inhabit, the future is full of rosy possibilities. Perhaps tomorrow we will sell that brilliant idea, or meet the person who will change our lives. Our culture stimulates these fantasies with constant images and stories of marvelous occurrences and happy romances.

The problem is, these images and fantasies exist only in our minds, or on-screen. They really aren't enough—we crave the real thing, not this endless daydreaming and titillation. Your task as a seducer is to bring some flesh and blood into someone's fantasy life by embodying a fantasy figure, or creating a scenario resembling that person's dreams. No one can resist the pull of a secret desire that has come to life before their eyes. You must first choose targets who have some repression or dream unrealized—always the most likely victims of a seduction. Slowly and gradually, you will build up the illusion that they are getting to see and feel and live those dreams of theirs. Once they have this sensation they will lose contact with reality, and begin to see your fantasy as more real than anything else. And once they lose touch with reality, they are (to quote Stendhal on Lord Byron's female victims) like roasted larks that fall into your mouth.

Most people have a misconception about illusion. As any magician knows, it need not be built out of anything grand or theatrical; the grand and theatrical can in fact be destructive, calling too much attention to you and your schemes. Instead create the appearance of normality. Once your targets feel secure—nothing is out of the ordinary—you have room to deceive them. In animating a fantasy, the great mistake is imagining it must be larger than life. That would border on camp, which is entertaining but rarely seductive. Instead, what you aim for is what Freud called the "uncanny," something strange and familiar at the same time, like a déjà vu, or a childhood memory—anything slightly irrational and dreamlike. The uncanny, the mix of the real and the unreal, has immense power over our imaginations. The fantasies you bring to life for your targets should not be bizarre or exceptional; they should be rooted in reality,

For this uncanny is in reality nothing new or alien, but something which is familiar and old—established in the mind and which has become alienated from it only through the process of repression. This reference to the factor of repression enables us, furthermore, to understand Schelling's definition of the uncanny as something which ought to have remained hidden but has come to light ...

• *...There is one more point of general application which I should like to add. . . . This is that an uncanny effect is often and easily produced when the distinction between imagination and reality is effaced,*

with a hint of the strange, the theatrical, the occult (in talk of destiny, for example). You vaguely remind people of something in their childhood, or a character in a film or book.

One night Pauline Bonaparte, the sister of Napoleon, held a gala affair in her house. Afterward, a handsome German officer approached her in the garden and asked for her help in passing along a request to the emperor. Pauline said she would do her best, and then, with a rather mysterious look in her eye, asked him to come back to the same spot the next night. The officer returned, and was greeted by a young woman who led him to some rooms near the garden and then to a magnificent salon, complete with an extravagant bath. Moments later, another young woman entered through a side door, dressed in the sheerest garments. It was Pauline. Bells were rung, ropes were pulled, and maids appeared, preparing the bath, giving the officer a dressing gown, then disappearing. The officer later described the evening as something out of a fairy tale, and he had the feeling that Pauline was deliberately acting the part of some mythical seductress. Part of the adventure was the feeling that she was playing a role, and was inviting the officer along into this shared fantasy.

Role playing is immensely pleasurable.

Its appeal goes back to childhood, where we first learn the thrill of trying on different parts, imitating adults or figures out of fiction. As we get older and society fixes a role on us, a part of us yearns for the playful approach we once had, the masks we were able to wear. We still want to play that game, to act a different role in life. Indulge your targets in this wish by first making it clear that you are playing a role, then inviting them to join you in a shared fantasy. The more you set things up like a play or a piece of fiction, the better.

When our emotions are engaged, we often have trouble seeing things as they are. Feelings of love cloud our vision, making us color events to coincide with our desires. To make people believe in the illusions you create, you need to feed the emotions over which they have least control. Often the best way to do this is to ascertain their unsatisfied desires, their wishes crying out for fulfillment. Perhaps they want to see themselves as noble or romantic, but life has thwarted them. Perhaps they want an adventure. If something seems to validate this wish, they become emotional and irrational, almost to the point of hallucination. Few have the power to see through an illusion they desperately want to believe in.

> *as when something that we have hitherto regarded as imaginary appears before us in reality, or when a symbol takes over the full functions of the thing it symbolizes, and so on. It is this factor which contributes not a little to the uncanny effect attaching to magical practices. The infantile element in this, which also dominates the minds of neurotics, is the overaccentuation of psychical reality in comparison with material reality—a feature closely allied to the belief in the omnipotence of thoughts.*
>
> —SIGMUND FREUD, "THE UNCANNY," IN *PSYCHOLOGICAL WRITINGS AND LETTERS*

Symbol: *Shangri-La. Everyone has a vision in their mind of a perfect place where people are kind and noble, where their dreams can be realized and their wishes fulfilled, where life is full of adventure and romance. Lead the target on a journey there, give them a glimpse of Shangri-La through the mists on the mountain, and they will fall in love.*

15
Isolate the Victim

*An iso-
lated person is weak. By
slowly isolating your victims, you
make them more vulnerable to your influence. Their isolation may be psychological: by filling their field of vision through the
pleasurable attention you pay them, you crowd
out everything else in their mind. They see and
think only of you. The isolation may also be physical: you take them away from their normal milieu,
friends, family, home. Give them the sense of being
marginalized, in limbo—they are leaving one world
behind and entering another. Once isolated like
this, they have no outside support, and in their
confusion they are easily led astray. Lure the
seduced into your lair, where nothing is
familiar.*

> *Put them in a spot where they have no place to go, and they will die before fleeing.*
>
> —SUN-TZU, THE ART OF WAR

Keys to Seduction

The people around you may seem strong, and more or less in control of their lives, but that is merely a facade. Underneath, people are more brittle than they let on. What lets them seem strong is the series of nests and safety nets they envelop themselves in—their friends, their families, their daily routines, which give them a feeling of continuity, safety, and control. Suddenly pull the rug out from under them, drop them alone into some foreign place where the familiar signposts are gone or scrambled, and you will see a very different person.

A target who is strong and settled is hard to seduce. But even the strongest people can be made vulnerable if you can isolate them from their nests and safety nets. Block out their friends and family with your constant presence, alienate them from the world they are used to, and take them to places they do not know. Get them to spend time in *your* environment. Deliberately disturb their habits, get them to do things they have never done. They will grow emotional, making it easier to lead them astray. Disguise all this in the form of a pleasurable experience, and your targets will wake up one day distanced from everything that normally comforts them. Then they will turn to you for help, like a child crying out for its mother when the lights are turned out. In seduction, as in warfare, the isolated target is weak and vulnerable.

Your worst enemies in a seduction are often your targets' family and friends. They are outside your circle and immune to your charms; they may provide a voice of reason to the seduced. You must work silently and subtly to alienate the target from them. Insinuate that they are jealous of your target's good fortune in finding you, or that they are parental figures who have lost a taste for adventure. The latter argument is extremely effective with young people, whose identities are in flux and who are more than ready to rebel against any authority figure, particularly their parents. You represent excitement and life; the friends and parents represent habit and boredom.

Our past attachments are a barrier to the present. Even people we have left behind can continue to have a hold on us. As a seducer you will be held up to the past, compared to previous suitors, perhaps found inferior. *Do not let it get to that point.* Crowd out the past with your attentions in the present. If necessary, find ways to disparage their previous lovers—subtly or not so subtly, depending on the situation. Even go so far as to open old wounds, making them feel old pain and seeing by contrast how much better the present is. The more you can isolate them from their past, the deeper they will sink with you into the present.

Many of us today are weighed down by all kinds of responsibilities. A wall forms around us—we are immune to the influence of other people, because we are so preoccupied. To seduce your targets, you need to lure them away, gently, slowly, from the affairs that fill their mind. And often what will best lure them from their castle walls is the whiff of the exotic. Offer something unfamiliar that will fascinate them and hold their attention. Be different in your manners and appearance, and slowly envelop them in this different world of yours. Do not worry that the disruption you represent is making them emotional—that is a sign of their growing weakness. Most people are ambivalent: on the one hand they feel comforted by their habits and duties, on the other they are bored, and ripe for anything that seems exotic, that seems to come from somewhere else. The deeper you lure them into your unfamiliar world, the more isolated they become. By the time they realize what has happened, it is too late.

The key to isolating your targets psychologically is to pay them intense attention, to make them feel that there is nothing

---

My child, my sister, dream \ How sweet all things would seem \ Were we in that kind land to live together, \ And there love slow and long, \ There love and die among \ Those scenes that image you, that sumptuous weather. \ Drowned suns that glimmer there \ Through cloud-dishevelled air \ Move me with such a mystery as appears \ Within those other skies \ Of your treacherous eyes \ When I behold them shining through their tears. \ There, there is nothing else but grace and measure, \ Richness, quietness, and pleasure ... \ See, sheltered from the swells \ There in the still canals \ Those else in the world but the two of you. You do not give them the time or space to worry about, suspect, or resist you; you flood them with the kind of attention that crowds out all other thoughts, concerns, and problems. This will have an intoxicating effect on their ego, and make them experience the isolation as something pleasurable.

The principle of isolation can be taken literally by whisking the target off to an exotic locale. The danger of travel is that your targets are intimately exposed to you—it is hard to maintain an air of mystery. But if you take them to a place alluring enough to distract them, you will prevent them from focusing on anything banal in your character.

The seductive power of isolation goes beyond the sexual realm. When new adherents joined Mahatma Gandhi's circle of devoted followers, they were encouraged to cut off their ties with the past—with their family and friends. This kind of renunciation has been a requirement of many religious sects over the centuries. People who isolate themselves in this way are much more vulnerable to influence and persuasion. A charismatic politician feeds off and even encourages people's feelings of alienation.

Finally, at some point in the seduction there must be a hint of danger in the mix.

> *drowsy ships that dream of sailing forth; \ It is to satisfy \ Your least desire, they ply \ Hither through all the waters of the earth. \ The sun at close of day \ Clothes the fields of hay, \ Then the canals, at last the town entire \ In hyacinth and gold: \ Slowly the land is rolled \ Sleepward under a sea of gentle fire. \ There, there is nothing else but grace and measure, \ Richness, quietness, and pleasure.*
>
> —CHARLES BAUDELAIRE, "INVITATION TO THE VOYAGE," *THE FLOWERS OF EVIL*, TRANSLATED BY RICHARD WILBUR

Your targets should feel that they are gaining a great adventure in following you, but are also losing something—a part of their past, their cherished comfort. Actively encourage these ambivalent feelings. An element of fear is the proper spice; although too much fear is debilitating, in small doses it makes us feel alive. Like diving out of an airplane, it is exciting, a thrill, at the same time that it is a little frightening. And the only person there to break the fall, or catch them, is you.

Symbol: *The Pied Piper. A jolly fellow in his red and yellow cloak, he lures the children from their homes with the delightful sounds of his flute. Enchanted, they do not notice how far they are walking, how they are leaving their families behind. They do not even notice the cave he eventually leads them into, and which closes upon them forever.*

16
Prove Yourself

Most people want to be seduced. If they resist your efforts, it is probably because you have not gone far enough to allay their doubts—about your motives, the depth of your feelings, and so on. One well-timed action that shows how far you are willing to go to win them over will dispel their doubts. Do not worry about looking foolish or making a mistake—any kind of deed that is self-sacrificing and for your targets' sake will so overwhelm their emotions, they won't notice anything else. Never appear discouraged by people's resistance, or complain. Instead, meet the challenge by doing something extreme or chivalrous. Conversely, spur others to prove themselves by making yourself hard to reach, unattainable, worth fighting over.

Love is a species of warfare. Slack troopers, go elsewhere! \ It takes more than cowards to guard \ These standards. Night-duty in winter, long-route marches, every \ Hardship, all forms of suffering: these await \ The recruit who expects a soft option. You'll often be out in \ Cloudbursts, and bivouac on the bare \ Ground ... Is lasting \ Love your ambition? Then put away all pride. \ The simple, straightforward way in may be denied you, \ Doors bolted, shut in your face — \ So be ready to slip down from the roof through a lightwell, \ Or sneak in by an upper-floor window. She'll be glad \ To know you're risking

Seductive Evidence

Anyone can talk big, say lofty things about their feelings, insist on how much they care for us, and also for all oppressed peoples in the far reaches of the planet. But if they never behave in a way that will back up their words, we begin to doubt their sincerity—perhaps we are dealing with a charlatan, or a hypocrite or a coward. Flattery and fine words can only go so far. A time will eventually arrive when you will have to show your victim some evidence, to match your words with deeds.

This kind of evidence has two functions. First, it allays any lingering doubts about you. Second, an action that reveals some positive quality in you is immensely seductive in and of itself. Brave or selfless deeds create a powerful and positive emotional reaction. Don't worry, your deeds do not have to be so brave and selfless that you lose everything in the process. The appearance alone of nobility will often suffice. In fact, in a world where people overanalyze and talk too much, any kind of action has a bracing, seductive effect.

It is normal in the course of a seduction to encounter resistance. The more obstacles you overcome, of course, the greater the pleasure that awaits you, but many a seduction fails because the seducer does not correctly read the resistances of the target. More often than not, you give up too easily. First, understand a primary law of seduction: resistance is a sign that the other person's emotions are engaged in the process. The only person you cannot seduce is somebody distant and cold. Resistance is emotional, and can be transformed into its opposite, much as, in jujitsu, the physical resistance of an opponent can be used to make him fall. If people resist you because they don't trust you, an apparently selfless deed, showing how far you are willing to go to prove yourself, is a powerful remedy. If they resist because they are virtuous, or because they are loyal to someone else, all the better—virtue and repressed desire are easily overcome by action. A chivalrous deed will also help eclipse any rivals on the scene, since most people are timid, and so rarely risk anything.

There are two ways to prove yourself. First, the spontaneous action: a situation arises in which the target needs help, a problem needs solving, or, simply, he or she needs a favor. You cannot foresee these situations, but you must be ready for them, for they can spring up at any time. Impress the target by going further than really necessary—sacrificing more money, more time, more effort than they had expected. Your

your neck, and for her sake: that will offer \Any mistress sure proof of your love.

—OVID, *THE ART OF LOVE*, TRANSLATED BY PETER GREEN

The man says: "... A fruit picked from one's own orchard ought to taste sweeter than one obtained from a stranger's tree, and what has been attained by greater effort is cherished more dearly than what is gained with little trouble. As the proverb says: 'Prizes great cannot be won unless some heavy labor's done.'" The woman says: "If no great prizes can be won unless some heavy labor's done, you must suffer the exhaustion of many toils to be able to attain the favors you seek, since what you ask for is a greater prize." The man says: "I give you all the thanks that I can express for so sagely promising me your love

target will often use these moments, or even manufacture them, as a kind of test: will you retreat? Or will you rise to the occasion? You cannot hesitate or flinch, even for a moment, or all is lost. If necessary, make the deed seem to have cost you more than it has, never with words, but indirectly—exhausted looks, reports spread through a third party, whatever it takes.

The second way to prove yourself is the brave deed that you plan and execute in advance, on your own and at the right moment—preferably some way into the seduction, when any doubts the victim still has about you are more dangerous than earlier on. Choose a dramatic, difficult action that reveals the painful time and effort involved. Danger can be extremely seductive. Cleverly lead your victim into a crisis, a moment of danger, or indirectly put them in an uncomfortable position, and you can play the rescuer, the gallant knight. The powerful feelings and emotions this elicits can easily be redirected into love.

Making your deed as dashing and chivalrous as possible will elevate the seduction to a new level, stir up deep emotions, and conceal any ulterior motives you may have. The sacrifices you are making must be visible; talking about them, or explaining what they have cost you, will seem like bragging. Lose sleep, fall ill, lose valuable time, put your career on the line, spend more money than you can afford. You can exaggerate all this for effect, but don't get caught boasting about it or feeling sorry for yourself: cause yourself pain and let them see it. Since almost everyone else in the world seems to have an angle, your noble and selfless deed will be irresistible.

Finally, this strategy can be applied in reverse by making people prove themselves to you. The heat of seduction is raised by such challenges—show me that you *really* love me. When one person (of either sex) rises to the occasion, often the other person is now expected to do the same, and the seduction heightens. By making people prove themselves, too, you raise your value and cover up your defects. Your targets are too busy trying to prove themselves to notice your blemishes and faults.

when I have performed great toils. God forbid that I or any other could win the love of so worthy a woman without first attaining it by many labors."

—ANDREAS CAPELLANUS ON LOVE, TRANSLATED BY P. G. WALSH

Symbol:

The Tournament. On the field, with its bright pennants and caparisoned horses, the lady looks on as knights fight for her hand. She has heard them declare love on bended knee, their endless songs and pretty promises. They are all good at such things. But then the trumpet sounds and the combat begins. In the tournament there can be no faking or hesitation. The knight she chooses must have blood on his face, and a few broken limbs.

17
Effect a Regression

*People who
have experienced a certain kind of
pleasure in the past will try to repeat or relive
it. The deepest-rooted and most pleasurable memories
are usually those from earliest childhood, and are often unconsciously associated with a parental figure. Bring your targets
back to that point by placing yourself in the oedipal triangle and
positioning them as the needy child. Unaware of the cause of their
emotional response, they will fall in love with you. Alternatively,
you too can regress, letting them play the role of the protecting,
nursing parent. In either case you are offering the ultimate
fantasy: the chance to have an intimate relationship
with mommy or daddy, son or daughter.*

The Erotic Regression

As adults we tend to overvalue our childhood. In their dependency and powerlessness, children genuinely suffer, yet when we get older we conveniently forget about that and sentimentalize the supposed paradise we have left behind. We forget the pain and remember only the pleasure. Why? Because the responsibilities of adult life are a burden so oppressive at times that we secretly yearn for the dependency of childhood, for that person who looked after our every need, assumed our cares and worries. This daydream of ours has a strong erotic component, for the child's feeling of being dependent on the parent is charged with sexual undertones. Give people a sensation similar to that protected, dependent feeling of childhood and they will project all kinds of fantasies onto you, including feelings of love or sexual attraction that they will attribute to something else. We won't admit it, but we long to regress, to shed our adult exterior and vent the childish emotions that linger beneath the surface.

To effect a regression you will need to encourage people to talk about their childhood. Most of us are only too happy to oblige; and our memories are so vivid and emotional that a part of us regresses just in talking about our early years. Also, in the course of talking,

> *I have stressed the fact that the beloved person is a substitute for the ideal ego. Two people who love each other are interchanging their ego-ideals. That they love each other means they love the ideal of themselves in the other one. There would be no love on earth if this phantom were not there. We fall in love because we cannot attain the image that is our better self and the best of our self. From this concept it is obvious that love itself is only possible on a certain cultural level or after a certain phase in the development of the personality has been reached. The creation of an ego-ideal itself marks human progress. When people are*

little secrets slip out: we reveal all kinds of valuable information about our weaknesses and our mental makeup, information you must attend to and remember. Do not take your targets' words at face value. Pay attention to their tone of voice, to any nervous tics as they talk, and particularly to anything they do not want to talk about, anything they deny or that makes them emotional. Many statements actually mean their opposite: should they say they hated their father, for instance, you can be sure that they are hiding a lot of disappointment—that they actually loved their father only too much, and perhaps never quite got what they wanted from him.

With the information you have gathered, you can now effect the regression. Perhaps you have uncovered a powerful attachment to a sibling, a teacher, or any early infatuation, a person who casts a shadow over their present lives. Knowing what it was about this person that affected them so powerfully, you can now take over that role. Or perhaps you have learned of an immense gap in their childhood—a neglectful father, for instance. You act like that parent now, but you replace the original neglect with the attention that the real parent never supplied.

The regressions you can effect fall into four main types.

entirely satisfied with their actual selves, love is impossible. • The transfer of the ego-ideal to a person is the most characteristic trait of love.

—THEODOR REIK,
OF LOVE AND LUST

EFFECT A REGRESSION | 151

The Infantile Regression. The first bond—the bond between a mother and her infant—is the most powerful one. Unlike other animals, human babies have a long period of helplessness during which they are dependent on their mother, creating an attachment that influences the rest of their lives. The key to effecting this regression is to reproduce the sense of unconditional love a mother has for her child. Never judge your targets—let them do whatever they want, including behaving badly; at the same time surround them with loving attention, smother them with comfort.

The Oedipal Regression. After the bond between mother and child comes the oedipal triangle of mother, father, and child. This triangle forms during the period of the child's earliest erotic fantasies. A boy wants his mother to himself, a girl does the same with her father, but they never quite have it that way, for a parent will always have competing connections to a spouse or to other adults. Unconditional love has gone; now, inevitably, the parent must sometimes deny what the child desires. Transport your victims back to this period. Play a parental role, be loving, but also sometimes scold and instill some discipline. Children actually love a little discipline—it makes them feel that the adult cares about them. And adult children too will be thrilled if you mix your tenderness with a little toughness and punishment.

Remember to include an erotic component in your parental behavior. Now your targets are not only getting their mother or father all to themselves, they are getting something more, something previously forbidden but now allowed.

The Ego Ideal Regression. As children, we often form an ideal figure out of our dreams and ambitions. First, that ideal figure is the person we want to be. We imagine ourselves as brave adventurers, romantic figures. Then, in our adolescence, we turn our attention to others, often projecting our ideals onto them. The first boy or girl we fall in love with may seem to have the ideal qualities we wanted for ourselves, or else may make us feel that we can play that ideal role in relation to them. Most of us carry these ideals around with us. We are secretly disappointed in how much we have had to compromise, how far below the ideal we have fallen as we have gotten older. Make your targets feel they are living out this youthful ideal, and coming closer to being the person they wanted to be, and you will effect a different kind of regression, creating a feeling reminiscent of adolescence. The relationship between you and the seduced is in this instance more equal than in the previous kinds of regressions—more like the affection between siblings. In fact the ideal is often modeled on a brother or sister. To create this effect, strive to reproduce the intense, innocent mood of a youthful infatuation.

The Reverse Parental Regression. Here you are the one to regress: you deliberately play the role of the cute, adorable, yet also sexually charged child. Older people always find younger people incredibly seductive. In the presence of youth, they feel a little of their own youth return; but they are in fact older, and mixed into the invigoration they feel in young people's company is the pleasure of playing the mother or father to them.

Symbol:
The Bed. Lying alone in bed, the child feels unprotected, afraid, and needy. In a nearby room, there is the parent's bed. It is large and forbidding, site of things you are not supposed to know about. Give the seduced both feelings—helplessness and transgression—as you lay them into bed and put them to sleep.

18
Stir Up the Transgressive and Taboo

There are always social limits on what one can do. Some of these, the most elemental taboos, go back centuries; others are more superficial, simply defining polite and acceptable behavior. Making your targets feel that you are leading them past either kind of limit is immensely seductive. People yearn to explore their dark side. Not everything in romantic love is supposed to be tender and soft; hint that you have a cruel, even sadistic streak. You do not respect age differences, marriage vows, family ties. Once the desire to transgress draws your targets to you, it will be hard for them to stop. Take them further than they imagined—the shared feeling of guilt and complicity will create a powerful bond.

Keys to Seduction

Hearts and eye go traveling along the paths that have always brought them joy; and if anyone attempts to spoil their game, he only makes them the more passionate about it, God knows ... so it was with Tristan and Isolde. As soon as they were forbidden their desires, and prevented from enjoying one another by spies and guards, they began to suffer intensely. Desire now seriously tormented them by its magic, many times worse than before; their need for one another was more painful and urgent than it had ever been. ... Women do lots of things just because they are forbidden, which they would certainly not

Society and culture are based on limits—this kind of behavior is acceptable, that is not. The limits are fluid and change with time, but there are always limits. The alternative is anarchy, the lawlessness of nature, which we dread. But we are strange animals: the moment any kind of limit is imposed, physically or psychologically, we are instantly curious. A part of us wants to go beyond that limit, to explore what is forbidden.

If, as children, we are told not to go past a certain point in the woods, that is precisely where we want to go. But we grow older, and become polite and deferential; more and more boundaries encumber our lives. Do not confuse politeness with happiness, however. It covers up frustration, unwanted compromise. How can we explore the shadow side of our personality without incurring punishment or ostracism? It seeps out in our dreams. We sometimes wake up with a sense of guilt at the murder, incest, adultery, and mayhem that goes on in our dreams, until we realize no one needs to know about it but ourselves. But give a person the sense that with you they will have a chance to explore the outer reaches of acceptable, polite behavior, that with you they can vent some of their closeted personality, and you create the ingredients for a deep and powerful seduction.

You will have to go beyond the point of merely teasing them with an elusive fantasy. The shock and seductive power will come from the reality of what you are offering them. If they have followed you merely out of curiosity, they may feel some fear and hesitation, but once they are hooked, they will find you hard to resist, for it is hard to return to a limit once you have transgressed and gone past it.

The moment people feel that something is prohibited, a part of them will want it. That is what makes a married man or woman such a delicious target—the more someone is prohibited, the greater the desire.

Since what is forbidden is desired, somehow you must make yourself seem forbidden. The most blatant way to do this is to engage in behavior that gives you a dark and forbidden aura. Theoretically you are someone to avoid; in fact you are too seductive to resist. Play up your dark side and you will have a similar effect. For your targets to be involved with you means going beyond their limits, doing something naughty and unacceptable—to society, to their peers. For many that is reason to bite the bait.

The great eighteenth-century rake the Duke de Richelieu had a predilection for

do if they were not forbidden ... Our Lord God gave Eve the freedom to do what she would with all the fruits, flowers, and plants there were in Paradise, except for only one, which he forbade her to touch on pain of death ... She took the fruit and broke God's commandment ... but it is my firm belief now that Eve would never have done this, if she had not been forbidden to.

—Gottfried von Strassburg, *Tristan und Isolde*, quoted in Andrea Hopkins, *The Book of Courtly Love*

Just lately I saw a tight-reined stallion / Get the bit in his teeth and bolt / Like lightning—yet the minute he felt the reins slacken, / Drop loose on his flying mane, / He stopped dead. We eternally chafe at restrictions, covet / Whatever's forbidden. (Look how a sick man who's told / No immersion hangs round the bathhouse.)... / Desire / Mounts for what's kept out of reach. A thief's attracted / By burglar-proof premises. How often will love / Thrive on a rival's approval? It's not your wife's beauty, but your own / Passion for her that gets us—she must / Have something, just to have hooked you. A girl locked up by her /

young girls and often he would heighten the seduction by enveloping them in transgressive behavior, to which the young are particularly susceptible. He would try to turn the young girl against her parents, ridiculing their religious zeal or prudery or pious behavior. The Duke's strategy was to attack the values that his targets held dearest—precisely the values that represent a limit. In a young person, family ties, religious ties, and the like are useful to the seducer; young people barely need a reason to rebel against them. The strategy, though, can be applied to a person of any age: for every deeply held value there is a shadow side, a doubt, a desire to explore what those values forbid.

Love is supposed to be tender and delicate, but in fact it can release violent and destructive emotions; and the possible violence of love, the way it breaks down our normal reasonableness, is just what attracts us. Approach romance's violent side by mixing a cruel streak into your tender attentions, particularly in the latter stages of the seduction, when the target is in your clutches. A masochistic involvement can represent a great transgressive release.

The more illicit your seduction feels, the more powerful its effect. Give your targets the feeling that they are committing a kind of crime, a deed whose guilt they share with you. Create public moments in which the two of you know something that those around you do not. It could be phrases and looks that only you recognize, a secret. It is critical to play on tensions like these in public, creating a sense of complicity and collusion against the world.

People may be straining to remove restrictions on private behavior, to make everything freer, in the world today, but that only makes seduction more difficult and less exciting. Do what you can to reintroduce a feeling of transgression and crime, even if it is only psychological or illusory. There must be obstacles to overcome, social norms to flout, laws to break, before the seduction can be consummated. It might seem that a permissive society imposes few limits; find some. There will always be limits, sacred cows, behavioral standards—endless ammunition for stirring up the transgressive and taboo.

Husband's not chaste but pursued, her fear's / A bigger draw than her figure. Illicit passion— like it / Or not—is sweeter. It only turns me on / When the girl says, "I'm frightened."

—OVID, THE AMORES, TRANSLATED BY PETER GREEN

Baseness attracts everybody.

—JOHANN WOLFGANG GOETHE

Symbol: The Forest. The children are told not to go into the forest that lies just beyond the safe confines of their home. There is no law there, only wilderness, wild animals, and criminals. But the chance to explore, the alluring darkness, and the fact that it is prohibited are impossible to resist. And once inside, they want to go farther and farther.

19
Use Spiritual Lures

Everyone has doubts and insecurities—about their body, their self-worth, their sexuality. If your seduction appeals exclusively to the physical, you will stir up these doubts and make your targets self-conscious. Instead, lure them out of their insecurities by making them focus on something sublime and spiritual: a religious experience, a lofty work of art, the occult. Play up your divine qualities; affect an air of discontent with worldly things; speak of the stars, destiny, the hidden threads that unite you and the object of the seduction. Lost in a spiritual mist, the target will feel light and uninhibited. Deepen the effect of your seduction by making its sexual culmination seem like the spiritual union of two souls.

Keys to Seduction

Religion is the most seductive system that mankind has created. Death is our greatest fear, and religion offers us the illusion that we are immortal, that something about us will live on. The idea that we are an infinitesimal part of a vast and indifferent universe is terrifying; religion humanizes this universe, makes us feel important and loved. We are not animals governed by uncontrollable drives, animals that die for no apparent reason, but creatures made in the image of a supreme being. We too can be sublime, rational, and good. Anything that feeds a desire or a wished-for illusion is seductive, and nothing can match religion in this arena.

Pleasure is the bait that you use to lure a person into your web. But no matter how clever a seducer you are, in the back of your targets' mind they are aware of the endgame, the physical conclusion toward which you are heading. You may think your target is unrepressed and hungry for pleasure, but almost all of us are plagued by an underlying unease with our animal nature. Unless you deal with this unease, your seduction, even when successful in the short term, will be superficial and temporary. Instead, try to capture your target's soul, to build the foundation of a deep and lasting seduction. Lure the victim deep into your web with spirituality, making physical pleasure seem sublime and transcendent. Spirituality will disguise your manipulations, suggesting that your relationship is timeless, and creating a space for ecstasy in the victim's mind. Remember that seduction is a mental process, and nothing is more mentally intoxicating than religion, spirituality, and the occult.

As a seducer, you use religion and spirituality as a kind of distracting device. You invite the other person to worship something beautiful in the world. It could be nature, a work of art, or an exotic religion. It could even be a noble cause, a saint or a guru. People are dying to believe in something. In the process your targets are taken outside themselves, connected to something larger, while distracted from the physical element of your seduction. If you can make yourself seem to resemble the thing you are worshipping—you are natural, aesthetic, noble, and sublime—your targets will transfer their worship to you. They will barely notice the transition to something more physical and sexual. From spiritual ecstasy to sexual ecstasy is but one small step.

Affect a spiritual air by displaying a discontent with the banalities of life. It is not money or sex or success that moves you;

The idealization of the [movie] star implies, of course, a corresponding spiritualization. Photographs often show us the star busy painting under the inspiration of the most authentic talent; or else crouching in front of his bookshelves to consult some handsome volume whose splendid binding guarantees the spiritual value. Ray Milland does not conceal the elevation of his preoccupations: "I love astronomy, I love thinking about nature and the possibility of life on other planets. My favorite book is about the vegetation that might exist on the moon ..." Love thus manufactured is evidently created in the image of love in the movies themselves: a passionate sentiment impregnated with spirituality. Of course the myth of the stars does not deny sexuality. Sexuality is always understood. The gossip columns imply it in their myriad "engagements" or "violent attractions." But the stars make love only as a result of a superior and desperate impulse of the soul. Priestesses of love, they transcend it in accomplishing it. They cannot give themselves up to debauch, i.e., to pleasure without spirituality, except under penalty of banishment from Beverly Hills. They must at

your drives are never so base. No, something much deeper motivates you. Whatever this is, keep it vague, letting the target imagine your hidden depths. The stars, astrology, fate, are always appealing; create the sense that destiny has brought you and your target together. That will make your seduction feel more natural. In a world where too much is controlled and manufactured, the sense that fate, necessity, or some higher power is guiding your relationship is doubly seductive. If you want to weave religious motifs into your seduction, it is always best to choose some distant, exotic religion with a slightly pagan air. It is easy to move from pagan spirituality to pagan earthiness. Timing counts: once you have stirred your targets' souls, move quickly to the physical, making sexuality seem merely an extension of the spiritual vibrations you are experiencing. In other words, employ the spiritual strategy as close to the time for your bold move as possible.

The spiritual is not exclusively the religious or the occult. It is anything that will add a sublime, timeless quality to your seduction. In the modern world, culture and art have in some ways taken the place of religion. There are two ways to use art in your seduction: first, create it yourself, in the target's honor. Poetry that they have inspired you to write will always work well.

Half Picasso's appeal to many women was the hope that he would immortalize them in his paintings—for *Ars longa, vita brevis* (Art is long, life is short), as they used to say in Rome. Even if your love is a passing fancy, by capturing it in a work of art you give it a seductive illusion of eternity. The second way to use art is to make it ennoble the affair, giving your seduction an elevated edge. Take your targets to the theater, to the opera, to museums, to places full of history and atmosphere. In such places your souls can vibrate to the same spiritual wavelength. Of course you should avoid works of art that are earthy or vulgar, calling attention to your intentions. The play, movie, or book can be contemporary, even a little raw, as long as it contains a noble message and is tied to some just cause. Even a political movement can be spiritually uplifting. Remember to tailor your spiritual lures to the target. If the target is earthy and cynical, paganism or art will be more productive than the occult or religious piety.

Spirituality, the love of God, is a sublimated version of sexual love. The language of the religious mystics of the Middle Ages is full of erotic images; the contemplation of God and of the sublime can offer a kind of mental orgasm. There is no more seductive brew than the combination of the spiritual

least pretend ... The star enjoys life and love on behalf of the whole world. She has the mystical greatness of the sacred prostitute.

—EDGAR MORIN,
THE STARS,
TRANSLATED BY
RICHARD HOWARD

and the sexual, the high and the low. When you talk of spiritual matters, then, let your looks and physical presence hint of sexuality at the same time. Make the harmony of the universe and union with God seem to confuse with physical harmony and the union between two people. If you can make the endgame of your seduction appear as a spiritual experience, you will heighten the physical pleasure and create a seduction with a deep and lasting effect.

Symbol:

The Stars in the sky. Objects of worship for centuries, and symbols of the sublime and divine. In contemplating them, we are momentarily distracted from everything mundane and mortal. We feel lightness. Lift your targets' minds up to the stars and they will not notice what is happening here on earth.

20
Mix Pleasure with Pain

The greatest mistake in seduction is being too nice. At first, perhaps, your kindness is charming, but it soon grows monotonous; you are trying too hard to please, and seem insecure. Instead of overwhelming your targets with niceness, try inflicting some pain. Lure them in with focused attention, then change direction, appearing suddenly uninterested. Make them feel guilty and insecure. Even instigate a breakup, subjecting them to an emptiness and pain that will give you room to maneuver—now a rapprochement, an apology, a return to your earlier kindness, will turn them weak at the knees. The lower the lows you create, the greater the highs. To heighten the erotic charge, create the excitement of fear.

> *The more one pleases generally, the less one pleases profoundly.*
>
> —STENDHAL, *LOVE*, TRANSLATED BY GILBERT AND SUZANNE SALE

Keys to Seduction

Almost everyone is more or less polite. We learn early on not to tell people what we really think of them; we smile at their jokes, act interested in their stories and problems. It is the only way to live with them. Eventually this becomes a habit; we are nice, even when it isn't really necessary. We try to please other people, to not step on their toes, to avoid disagreements and conflict.

Niceness in seduction, however, though it may at first draw someone to you (it is soothing and comforting), soon loses all effect. Being too nice can literally push the target away from you. Erotic feeling depends on the creation of tension. Without tension, without anxiety and suspense, there can be no feeling of release, of true pleasure and joy. It is your task to create that tension in the target, to stimulate feelings of anxiety, to lead them to and fro, so that the culmination of the seduction has real weight and intensity. So rid yourself of your nasty habit of avoiding conflict, which is in any case unnatural. You are most often nice not out of your own inner goodness but out of fear of displeasing, out of insecurity. Go beyond that fear and you suddenly have options— the freedom to create pain, then magically dissolve it. Your seductive powers will increase tenfold.

People will be less upset by your hurtful actions than you might imagine. In the world today, we often feel starved for experience. We crave emotion, even if it is negative. The pain you cause your targets, then, is bracing—it makes them feel more alive. They have something to complain about, they get to play the victim. As a result, once you have turned the pain into pleasure they will readily forgive you. Stir up their jealousy, make them feel insecure, and the validation you later give their ego by preferring them over their rivals is doubly delightful. Remember: you have more to fear by boring your targets than by shaking them up. Wounding people binds them to you more deeply than kindness. If you need inspiration, find the part of the target that most irritates you and use it as a springboard for some therapeutic conflict. The more real your cruelty, the more effective it is.

There is something bracing about fear. It makes you vibrate with sensation, heightens your awareness, is intensely erotic. The closer you bring your targets to the edge of the precipice, to the feeling that you could abandon them, the dizzier and more lost they will become. Falling in love means literally falling—losing control, a mix of fear and excitement.

> *"Certainly," I said, "I have often told you that pain holds a peculiar attraction for me, and that nothing kindles my passion quite so much as tyranny, cruelty and above all unfaithfulness in a beautiful woman."*
>
> —LEOPOLD VON SACHER-MASOCH, *VENUS IN FURS*, TRANSLATED BY JEAN MCNEIL

Oderint, dum metuant [Let them hate me so long as they fear me], as if only fear and hate belong together, whereas fear and love have nothing to do with each other, as if it were not fear that makes love interesting. With what kind of love do we embrace nature? Is there not a secretive anxiety and horror in it, because its beautiful harmony works its way out of lawlessness and wild confusion, its security out of perfidy? But precisely this anxiety captivates the most. So also with love, if it is to be interesting. Behind it ought to brood the deep, anxious night from which springs the flower of love.

—SÖREN KIERKEGAARD, THE

Never let your targets get too comfortable with you. They need to feel anxiety. Show them some coldness, a flash of anger they did not expect. Be irrational if necessary. There is always the trump card: a breakup. Let them feel they have lost you forever, make them fear that they have lost the power to charm you. Let these feelings sit with them for a while, then pull them back from the precipice. The reconciliation will be intense.

Many of us have masochistic yearnings without realizing it. It takes someone to inflict some pain on us for these deeply repressed desires to come to the surface. You must learn to recognize the types of hidden masochists out there, for each one enjoys a particular kind of pain. For instance, there are people who feel that they deserve nothing good in life, and who, unable to deal with success, sabotage themselves constantly. Be nice to them, admit that you admire them, and they are uncomfortable, since they feel that they cannot possibly match up to the ideal figure you have clearly imagined them to be. Such self-saboteurs do better with a little punishment; scold them, make them aware of their inadequacies. They feel they deserve such criticism and when it comes it is with a sense of relief. It is also easy to make them feel guilty, a feeling that deep down they enjoy.

Other people experience the responsibilities and duties of modern life as such a heavy burden, they long to give it all up. These people are often looking for someone or something to worship—a cause, a religion, a guru. Make them worship you. And then there are those who want to play the martyr. Recognize them by the joy they take in complaining, in feeling righteous and wronged; then give them a reason to complain. Remember: appearances deceive. Often the strongest-looking people may secretly want to be punished. In any event, follow up pain with pleasure and you will create a state of dependency that will last for a long time.

As a seducer you must find a way to lower people's resistances. The Charmer's approach of flattery and attention can be effective, particularly with the insecure, but it can take months of work, and can also backfire. To get a quicker result, and to break down more inaccessible people, it is often better to alternate harshness and kindness. By being harsh you create inner tensions—your targets may be upset with you, but they are also asking themselves questions. What have they done to earn your dislike? When you then are kind, they

Seducer's Diary,
translated by
Howard V. Hong
and Edna H. Hong

In essence, the domain of eroticism is the domain of violence, of violation ... The whole business of eroticism is to strike to the inmost core of the living being, so that the heart stands still ... The whole business of eroticism is to destroy the self-contained character of the participators as they are in their normal lives ... We ought never to forget that in spite of the bliss love promises its first effect is one of turmoil and distress. Passion fulfilled itself provokes such violent agitation that the

> *happiness involved, before being a happiness to be enjoyed, is so great as to be more like its opposite, suffering ... The likelihood of suffering is all the greater since suffering alone reveals the total significance of the beloved object.*
>
> —GEORGES BATAILLE, *EROTISM: DEATH AND SENSUALITY*, TRANSLATED BY MARY DALWOOD

feel relieved, but also concerned that at any moment they might somehow displease you again. Make use of this pattern to keep them in suspense—dreading your harshness and keen to keep you kind.

Finally, your seduction should never follow a simple course upward toward pleasure and harmony. The climax will come too soon, and the pleasure will be weak. What makes us intensely appreciate something is previous suffering. A brush with death makes us fall in love with life; a long journey makes a return home that much more pleasurable. Your task is to create moments of sadness, despair, and anguish, to create the tension that allows for a great release. Do not worry about making people angry; anger is a sure sign that you have your hooks in them. Nor should you be afraid that if you make yourself difficult people will flee—we only abandon those who bore us. The ride on which you take your victims can be tortuous but never dull. At all costs, keep your targets emotional and on edge. Create enough highs and lows and you will wear away the last vestiges of their willpower.

Symbol: *The Precipice. At the edge of a cliff, people often feel lightheaded, both fearful and dizzy. For a moment they can imagine themselves falling headlong. At the same time, a part of them is tempted. Lead your targets as close to the edge as possible, then pull them back. No thrill without fear.*

21
Give Them Space to Fall— The Pursuer is Pursued

If your targets become too used to you as the aggressor, they will give less of their own energy, and the tension will slacken. You need to wake them up, turn the tables. Once they are under your spell, take a step back and they will start to come after you. Begin with a touch of aloofness, an unexpected nonappearance, a hint that you are growing bored. Stir the pot by seeming interested in someone else. Make none of this explicit; let them only sense it and their imagination will do the rest, creating the doubt you desire. Soon they will want to possess you physically, and restraint will go out the window. The goal is to have them fall into your arms of their own will. Create the illusion that the seducer is being seduced.

Keys to Seduction

Since humans are naturally obstinate and willful creatures, and prone to suspicions of people's motives, it is only natural, in the course of any seduction, that in some ways your target will resist you. Seductions, then, are rarely easy or without setbacks. But once your victims overcome some of their doubts, and begin to fall under your spell, they will reach a point where they start to let go. They may sense that you are leading them along, but they are enjoying it. No one likes things to be complicated and difficult, and your target will expect the conclusion to come quickly. That is the point, however, where you must train yourself to hold back. Deliver the pleasurable climax they are so greedily awaiting, succumb to the natural tendency to bring the seduction to a rapid end, and you will have missed an opportunity to ratchet up the tension, to make the affair more heated. After all, you don't want a passive little victim to toy with; you want the seduced to engage their will in all its force, to become active participants in the seduction. You want them to pursue you, hopelessly ensnaring themselves in your web in the process. The only way to accomplish this is to take a step back and make them anxious.

You have strategically retreated before

Omissions, denials, deflections, deceptions, diversions, and humility—all aimed at provoking this second state, the secret of true seduction. Vulgar seduction might proceed by persistence, but true seduction proceeds by absence ... It is like fencing: one needs a field for the feint. Throughout this period, the seducer [Johannes], far from seeking to close in on her, seeks to maintain his distance by various ploys: he does not speak directly to her but only to her aunt, and then about trivial or stupid subjects; he neutral-izes everything by irony and feigned pedanticism; he fails to respond to

> *any feminine or erotic movement, and even finds her a sitcom suitor to disenchant and deceive her, to the point where she herself takes the initiative and breaks off her engagement, thus completing the seduction and creating the ideal situation for her total abandon.*
>
> —JEAN BAUDRILLARD, *SEDUCTION*, TRANSLATED BY BRIAN SINGER

(see chapter 12), but this is different. The target is falling for you now, and your retreat will lead to panicky thoughts: you are losing interest, it is somehow my fault, perhaps it is something I have done. Rather than think you are rejecting them on your own, your targets will want to make this interpretation, since if the cause of the problem is something they have done, they have the power to win you back by changing their behavior. If you are simply rejecting them, on the other hand, they have no control. People always want to preserve hope. Now they will come to you, turn aggressive, thinking that will do the trick. They will raise the erotic temperature. Understand: a person's willpower is directly linked to their libido, their erotic desire. When your victims are passively waiting for you, their erotic level is low. When they turn pursuer, getting involved in the process, brimming with tension and anxiety, the temperature is raised. So raise it as high as you can.

When you withdraw, make it subtle; you are instilling unease. Your coldness or distance should dawn on your targets when they are alone, in the form of a poisonous doubt creeping into their mind. Their paranoia will become self-generating. Your subtle step back will make them want to possess you, so they will willingly advance into your arms without being pushed. This is different from the strategy in chapter 20, in which you are inflicting deep wounds, creating a pattern of pain and pleasure. There the goal is to make your victims weak and dependent, here it is to make them active and aggressive. Which strategy you prefer to use (the two cannot be combined) depends on what you want and the proclivities of your victim.

Each gender has its own seductive lures, which come naturally to them. When you seem interested in someone but do not respond sexually, it is disturbing, and presents a challenge: they will find a way to seduce you. To produce this effect, first reveal an interest in your targets, through letters or subtle insinuation. But when you are in their presence, assume a kind of sexless neutrality. Be friendly, even warm, but no more. You are pushing them into arming themselves with the seductive charms that are natural to their sex—exactly what you want.

In the latter stages of the seduction, let your targets feel that you are becoming interested in another person—this is another form of taking a step back. When Napoleon Bonaparte first met the young widow Josephine de Beauharnais in 1795, he felt excited by her exotic beauty and the

> *I retreat and thereby teach her to be victorious as she pursues me. I continually fall back, and in this backward movement I teach her to know through me all the powers of erotic love, its turbulent thoughts, its passion, what longing is, and hope, and impatient expectancy.*
>
> —SÖREN KIERKEGAARD, *THE SEDUCER'S DIARY*

looks she gave him. He began to attend her weekly soirées and to his delight, she would ignore the other men and remain at his side, listening to him so attentively. He found himself falling in love with Josephine, and had every reason to believe she felt the same.

Then, at one soirée, she was friendly and attentive, as usual—except that she was equally friendly to another man there, a former aristocrat, like Josephine, the kind of man that Napoleon could never compete with when it came to manners and wit. Doubts and jealousies began to stir within. As a military man, he knew the value of going on the offensive, and after a few weeks of a swift and aggressive campaign he had her all to himself, eventually marrying her. Of course Josephine, a clever seductress, had set it all up. She did not say she was interested in another man, but his mere presence at her house, a look here and there, subtle gestures, made it seem that way. There is no more powerful way to hint that you are losing your desire. Make your interest in another too obvious, though, and it could backfire. This is not the situation in which you want to seem cruel; doubt and anxiety are the effects you are after. Make your possible interest in another barely perceptible to the naked eye.

Once someone has fallen for you, any physical absence will create unease. You are literally creating space. Your absences at this latter point of the seduction should seem at least somewhat justified. You are insinuating not a blatant brush-off but a slight doubt: perhaps you could have found some reason to stay, perhaps you are losing interest, perhaps there is someone else. In your absence, their appreciation of you will grow. They will forget your faults, forgive your sins. The moment you return, they will chase after you as you desire. It will be as if you had come back from the dead.

According to the psychologist Theodor Reik, we learn to love only through rejection. As infants, we are showered with love by our mother—we know nothing else. But when we get a little older, we begin to sense that her love is not unconditional. If we do not behave, if we do not please her, she can withdraw it. The idea that she will withdraw her affection fills us with anxiety, and, at first, with anger—we will show her, we will throw a tantrum. But that never works, and we slowly realize that the only way to keep her from rejecting us again is to imitate her—to be as loving, kind, and affectionate as she is. This will bond her to us in the deepest way. The pattern is ingrained in us for the rest of our lives: by experiencing a rejection or a coldness, we learn to court and pursue, to love.

Re-create this primal pattern in your seduction. First, shower your targets with affection. They will not be sure where this is coming from, but it is a delightful feeling, and they will never want to lose it. When it does go away, in your strategic step back, they will have moments of anxiety and anger, perhaps throwing a tantrum, and then the same childlike reaction: the only way to win you back, to have you for sure, will be to reverse the pattern, to imitate you, to be the affectionate, giving one. It is the terror of rejection that turns the tables.

This pattern will often repeat itself naturally in an affair or relationship. One person goes cold, the other pursues, then goes cold in turn, making the first person the pursuer, and on and on. As a seducer, do not leave this to chance. Make it happen. You are teaching the other person to become a seducer, just as the mother in her own way taught the child to return her love by turning her back. For your own sake learn to relish this reversal of roles. Do not merely play at being the pursued, but enjoy it, give in to it. The pleasure of being pursued by your victim can often surpass the thrill of the hunt.

Symbol: *The Pomegranate. Carefully cultivated and tended, the pomegranate begins to ripen. Do not gather it too early or force it off the stem—it will be hard and bitter. Let the fruit grow heavy and full of juice, then stand back—it will fall on its own. That is when its pulp is most delicious.*

22
Use Physical Lures

Targets with active minds are dangerous: if they see through your manipulations, they may suddenly develop doubts. Put their minds gently to rest, and waken their dormant senses, by combining a nondefensive attitude with a charged sexual presence. While your cool, nonchalant air is calming their minds and lowering their inhibitions, your glances, voice, and bearing—oozing sex and desire—are getting under their skin, agitating their senses and raising their temperature. Never force the physical; instead infect your targets with heat, lure them into lust. Lead them into the moment—an intensified present in which morality, judgment, and concern for the future all melt away and the body succumbs to pleasure.

Keys to Seduction

Now more than ever, our minds are in a state of constant distraction, barraged with endless information, pulled in every direction. Many of us recognize the problem: articles are written, studies are completed, but they simply become more information to digest. It is almost impossible to turn off an overactive mind; the attempt simply triggers more thoughts—an inescapable hall of mirrors. Perhaps we turn to alcohol, to drugs, to physical activity—anything to help us slow the mind, be more present in the moment. Our discontent presents the crafty seducer with infinite opportunity. The waters around you are teeming with people seeking some kind of release from mental overstimulation. The lure of unencumbered physical pleasure will make them take your bait, but as you prowl the waters, understand: the only way to relax a distracted mind is to make it focus on one thing. A hypnotist asks the patient to focus on a watch swinging back and forth. Once the patient focuses, the mind relaxes, the senses awaken, the body becomes prone to all kinds of novel sensations and suggestions. As a seducer, you are a hypnotist, and what you are making the target focus on is you.

Throughout the seductive process you

> CÉLIE: *What is the moment, and how do you define it? Because I must say in all good honesty that I do not understand you.* • THE DUKE: *A certain disposition of the senses, as unexpected as it is involuntary, which a woman can conceal, but which, should it be perceived or sensed by someone who might profit from it, puts her in the greatest danger of being a little more willing than she thought she ever should or could be.*
>
> —CRÉBILLON FILS, *LE HASARD AU COIN DU FEU*, QUOTED IN MICHEL FEHER, ED., *THE LIBERTINE READER*

When, on an autumn evening, with closed eyes, \ I breathe the warm dark fragrance of your *breast, \ Before me blissful shores unfold, caressed \ By dazzling fires from blue unchanging skies. \And there, upon that calm and drowsing isle, \ Grow luscious fruits amid fantastic trees: \ There, men are lithe: the women of those seas \ Amaze one with their gaze that knows no guile. \ Your perfume wafts me thither like a wind: \ I see a harbor thronged with masts and sails \ Still weary from the tumult of the gales; \ And with the sailors' song that drifts to me \ Are mingled odors of the tamarind, \ —And all my soul is scent and melody.*

—CHARLES BAUDELAIRE, "EXOTIC PERFUME," THE FLOWERS OF EVIL, TRANSLATED BY ALAN CONDER

have been filling the target's mind. Letters, mementos, shared experiences keep you constantly present, even when you are not there. Now, as you shift to the physical part of the seduction, you must see your targets more often. Your attention must become more intense. The more your targets think of you, the less they are distracted by thoughts of work and duty. When the mind focuses on one thing it relaxes, and when the mind relaxes, all the little paranoid thoughts that we are prone to—do you really like me, am I intelligent or beautiful enough, what does the future hold—vanish from the surface. Remember: it all starts with you. Be undistracted, present in the moment, and the target will follow suit. The intense gaze of the hypnotist creates a similar reaction in the patient.

Once the target's overactive mind starts to slow down, their senses will come to life, and your physical lures will have double their power. You will have a tendency to employ physical lures that work primarily on the eyes, the sense we most rely on in our culture. Physical appearances are critical, but you are after a general agitation of the senses. The senses are interconnected—an appeal to smell will trigger touch, an appeal to touch will trigger vision: casual or "accidental" contact—better a brushing of the skin than something more forceful right now—will create a jolt and activate the eyes. Subtly modulate the voice, make it slower and deeper. Living senses will crowd out rational thought.

During the seduction, you will have had to hold yourself back, to intrigue and frustrate the victim. You will have frustrated yourself in the process, and will already be champing at the bit. Once you sense that the target has fallen for you and cannot turn back, let those frustrated desires course through your blood and warm you up. Sexual desire is contagious. They will catch your heat and glow in return.

The seducer leads the victim to a point where he or she reveals involuntary signs of physical excitation that can be read in various symptoms. Once those signs are detected, the seducer must work quickly, applying pressure on the target to get lost in the moment—the past, the future, all moral scruples vanishing in air. Once your victims lose themselves in the moment, it is all over—their mind, their conscience, no longer holds them back. The body gives in to pleasure.

In leading your victims into the moment, remember a few things. First, a disordered look (tousled hair, ruffled dress) has more effect on the senses than a neat

A sweet disorder in the dress \ Kindles in clothes a wantonness: \ A lawn about the shoulders thrown \ Into a fine distraction: \ An erring lace, which here and there \ Enthralls the crimson stomacher: \ A cuff neglectful, and thereby \ Ribbands to flow confusedly: \ A winning wave (deserving note) \ In the tempestuous petticoat: \ A careless shoestring, in whose tie \ I see a wild civility: \ Do more bewitch me, than when art \ Is too precise in every part.

—ROBERT HERRICK, "DELIGHT IN DISORDER," QUOTED IN PETER WASHINGTON, ED., EROTIC POEMS appearance. It suggests the bedroom. Second, be alert to the signs of physical excitation. Blushing, trembling of the voice, tears, unusually forceful laughter, relaxing movements of the body (any kind of involuntary mirroring, their gestures imitating yours), a revealing slip of the tongue—these are signs that the victim is slipping into the moment and pressure is to be applied.

Seduction, like warfare, is often a game of distance and closeness. At first you track your enemy from a distance. Once the victim is heated up, you quickly bridge the distance, turning to hand-to-hand combat in which you give the enemy no room to withdraw, no time to think or to consider the position in which you have placed him or her. To take the element of fear out of this, use flattery, make the target feel more masculine or feminine, praise their charms. It is *their* fault that you have become so physical and aggressive. There is no greater physical lure than to make the target feel alluring.

Shared physical activity—swimming, dancing, sailing—is always an excellent lure. In such activity, the mind turns off and the body operates according to its own laws. The target's body will follow your lead, will mirror your moves, as far as you want it to go.

In the moment, all moral considerations fade away, and the body returns to a state of innocence. You can partly create that feeling through a devil-may-care attitude. When the time comes to make the seduction physical, train yourself to let go of your own inhibitions, your doubts, your lingering feelings of guilt and anxiety. Your confidence and ease will have more power to intoxicate the victim than all the alcohol you could apply. Exhibit a lightness of spirit—nothing bothers you, nothing daunts you, you take nothing personally. Do not talk of work, duty, marriage, the past or future. Plenty of other people will do that. Do not worry about what people think of you; do not judge your targets in any way. You are drawing them into an adventure, free of society's strictures and moral judgments. With you they can act out a fantasy—which, for many, might be the chance to be aggressive or transgressive, to experience danger. So empty yourself of your tendency to moralize and judge. You have lured your targets into a momentary world of pleasure—soft and accommodating, all rules and taboos thrown out the window.

Symbol: *The Raft. Floating out to sea, drifting with the current. Soon the shoreline disappears from sight, and the two of you are alone. The water invites you to forget all cares and worries, to submerge yourself. Without anchor or direction, cut off from the past, you give in to the drifting sensation and slowly lose all restraint.*

23
Master the Art of the Bold Move

A moment has arrived:
your victim clearly desires you, but is not ready
to admit it openly, let alone act on it. This is the time
to throw aside chivalry, kindness, and coquetry and to
overwhelm with a bold move. Don't give the victim time to
consider the consequences; create conflict, stir up tension,
so that the bold move comes as a great release. Showing
hesitation or awkwardness means you are thinking of
yourself, as opposed to being overwhelmed by the victim's
charms. Never hold back or meet the target halfway, under
the belief that you are being correct and considerate; you
must be seductive now, not political. One person must go
on the offensive, and it is you.

> *The more timidity a lover shows with us the more it concerns our pride to goad him on; the more respect he has for our resistance, the more respect we demand of him. We would willingly say to you men: "Ah, in pity's name do not suppose us to be so very virtuous; you are forcing us to have too much of it."*
>
> —Ninon de l'Enclo

Keys to Seduction

Think of seduction as a world you enter, a world that is separate and distinct from the real world. The rules are different here; what works in daily life can have the opposite effect in seduction. The real world features a democratizing, leveling impulse, in which everything has to seem at least something like equal. An overt imbalance of power, an overt desire for power, will stir envy and resentment; we learn to be kind and polite, at least on the surface. Even those who have power generally try to act humble and modest—they do not want to offend. In seduction, on the other hand, you can throw all of that out, revel in your dark side, inflict a little pain—in some ways be more yourself. Your naturalness in this respect will prove seductive in itself. The problem is that after years of living in the real world, we lose the ability to be ourselves. We become timid, humble, overpolite. Your task is to regain some of your childhood qualities, to root out all this false humility. And the most important quality to recapture is boldness.

No one is born timid; timidity is a protection we develop. If we never stick our necks out, if we never try, we will never have to suffer the consequences of failure or success. If we are kind and unobtrusive, no one will be offended—in fact we will seem saintly and likable. In truth, timid people are often self-absorbed, obsessed with the way people see them, and not at all saintly. And humility may have its social uses, but it is deadly in seduction. You need to be able to play the humble saint at times; it is a mask you wear. But in seduction, take it off. Boldness is bracing, erotic, and absolutely necessary to bring the seduction to its conclusion. Done right, it tells your targets that they have made you lose your normal restraint, and gives them license to do so as well. People are yearning to have a chance to play out the repressed sides of their personality. At the final stage of a seduction, boldness eliminates any awkwardness or doubts.

In a dance, two people cannot lead. One takes over, sweeping the other along. Seduction is not egalitarian; it is not a harmonic convergence. Holding back at the end out of fear of offending, or thinking it correct to share the power, is a recipe for disaster. This is an arena not for politics but for pleasure. It can be by the man or woman, but a bold move is required. If you are so concerned about the other person, console yourself with the thought that the pleasure of the one who surrenders is often greater than that of the aggressor.

A man should proceed to enjoy any woman when she gives him an opportunity and makes her own love manifest to him by the following signs: she calls out to a man without first being addressed by him; she shows herself to him in secret places; she speaks to him tremblingly and inarticulately; her face blooms with delight and her fingers or toes perspire; and sometimes she remains with both hands placed on his body as if she had been surprised by something, or as if overcome with fatigue. • After a woman has manifested her love to him by outward signs, and by the motions of her body, the man should make every possible attempt to conquer her. There should be no indecision or hesitancy: if an opening is found the man should make the most of it. The woman, indeed, becomes disgusted with the man if he is timid about his chances and throws them away. Boldness is the rule, for everything is to be gained, and nothing lost.

—THE HINDU ART OF LOVE, COLLECTED AND EDITED BY EDWARD WINDSOR

The bold move should come as a pleasant surprise, but not too much of a surprise. Learn to read the signs that the target is falling for you. His or her manner toward you will have changed—it will be more pliant, with more words and gestures mirroring yours—yet there will still be a touch of nervousness and uncertainty. Inwardly they have given in to you, but they do not expect a bold move. This is the time to strike. If you wait too long, to the point where they consciously desire and expect you to make a move, it loses the piquancy of coming as a surprise. You want a degree of tension and ambivalence, so that the move represents a great release. Their surrender will relieve tension like a long-awaited summer storm. Don't plan your bold move in advance; it cannot seem calculated. Wait for the opportune moment.

Be attentive to favorable circumstances. This will give you room to improvise and go with the moment, which will heighten the impression you want to create of being suddenly overwhelmed by desire. If you ever sense that the victim is expecting the bold move, take a step back, lull them into a false sense of security, then strike.

Your bold move should have a theatrical quality to it. That will make it memorable, and make your aggressiveness seem pleasant, part of the drama. The theatricality can come from the setting—an exotic or sensual location. It can also come from your actions. An element of fear—someone might find you, say—will heighten the tension. Remember: you are creating a moment that must stand out from the sameness of daily life.

Keeping your targets emotional will both weaken them and heighten the drama of the moment. And the best way to keep them at an emotional pitch is by infecting them with emotions of your own. People are very susceptible to the moods of those around them; this is particularly acute at the latter stages of a seduction, when resistance is low and the target has fallen under your spell. At the point of the bold move, learn to infect your target with whatever emotional mood you require, as opposed to suggesting the mood with words. You want access to the target's unconscious, which is best obtained by infecting them with emotions, bypassing their conscious ability to resist.

It may seem expected for the male to make the bold move, but history is full of successfully bold females. There are two main forms of feminine boldness. In the first, more traditional form, the coquettish woman stirs male desire, is completely in control, then at the last minute, after bringing her victim to a boil, steps back and lets him make the bold move. She sets it up, then signals with her eyes, her gestures, that she is ready for him. Courtesans have used this method throughout history. This lets the man maintain his masculine illusions, although the woman is really the aggressor.

The second form of feminine boldness does not bother with such illusions: the woman simply takes charge, initiates the first kiss, pounces on her victim. Many men find it not emasculating at all but very exciting. It all depends on the insecurities and proclivities of the victim. This kind of feminine boldness has its allure because it is more rare than the first kind, but then all boldness is somewhat rare. A bold move will always stand out compared to the usual treatment afforded by the tepid husband, the timid lover, the hesitant suitor. That is how you want it. If everyone were bold, boldness would quickly lose its allure.

Symbol:

The Summer Storm. The hot days follow one another, with no end in sight. The earth is parched and dry. Then there comes a stillness in the air, thick and oppressive—the calm before the storm. Suddenly gusts of wind arrive, and flashes of lightning, exciting and frightening. Allowing no time to react or run for shelter, the rain comes, and brings with it a sense of release. At last.

24
Beware the Aftereffects

*Danger follows
in the aftermath of a successful seduction. After emotions have reached a pitch,
they often swing in the opposite direction—toward
lassitude, distrust, disappointment. Beware of the long,
drawn-out goodbye; insecure, the victim will cling and claw,
and both sides will suffer. If you are to part, make the sacrifice
swift and sudden. If necessary, deliberately break the spell you
have created. If you are to stay in a relationship, beware a flag-
ging of energy, a creeping familiarity that will spoil the
fantasy. If the game is to go on, a second seduction is
required. Never let the other person take you for
granted—use absence, create pain and conflict, to keep the seduced on ten-
terhooks.*

Disenchantment

Seduction is a kind of spell, an *enchantment*. When you seduce, you are not quite your normal self; your presence is heightened, you are playing more than one role, you are strategically concealing your tics and insecurities. You have deliberately created mystery and suspense to make the victim experience a real-life drama. Under your spell, the seduced gets to feel transported away from the world of work and responsibility.

You will keep this going for as long as you want or can, heightening the tension, stirring the emotions, until the time finally comes to complete the seduction. After that, *disenchantment* almost inevitably sets in. The release of tension is followed by a letdown—of excitement, of energy—that can even materialize as a kind of disgust directed at you by your victim, even though what is happening is really a natural emotional course. It is as if a drug were wearing off, allowing the target to see you as you are—and being disappointed by the flaws that are inevitably there. On your side, you too have probably tended to idealize your targets somewhat, and once your desire is satisfied, you may see them as weak. (After all, they have given in to you.) You too may feel disappointed. Even in the best of circumstances, you are dealing

In a word, woe to the woman of too monotonous a temperament; her monotony satiates and disgusts. She is always the same statue, with her a man is always right. She is so good, so gentle, that she takes away from people the privilege of quarreling with her, and this is often such a great pleasure! Put in her place a vivacious woman, capricious, decided, to a certain limit, however, and things assume a different aspect. The lover will find in the same person the pleasure of variety. Temper is the salt, the quality which prevents it from becoming stale. Restlessness, jealousy, quarrels, making friends again,

> *spitefulness, all are the food of love. Enchanting variety? ... Too constant a peace is productive of a deadly ennui. Uniformity kills love, for as soon as the spirit of method mingles in an affair of the heart, the passion disappears, languor supervenes, weariness begins to wear, and disgust ends the chapter.*
>
> —Ninon de l'Enclos, Life, Letters and Epicurean Philosophy of Ninon de l'Enclos

now with the reality rather than the fantasy, and the flames will slowly die down—unless you start up a second seduction.

You may think that if the victim is to be sacrificed, none of this matters. But sometimes your effort to break off the relationship will inadvertently revive the spell for the other person, causing him or her to cling to you tenaciously. No, in either direction—sacrifice, or the integration of the two of you into a couple—you must take disenchantment into account. There is an art to the post-seduction as well.

Master the following tactics to avoid undesired aftereffects.

Fight against inertia. The sense that you are trying less hard is often enough to disenchant your victims. Reflecting back on what you did during the seduction, they will see you as manipulative: you wanted something then, and so you worked at it, but now you are taking them for granted. After the first seduction is over, then, show that it isn't really over—that you want to keep proving yourself, focusing your attention on them, luring them.

Often the best way to keep them enchanted is to inject intermittent drama. This can be painful—opening old wounds, stirring up jealousy, withdrawing a little. On the other hand it can also be pleasant: think about proving yourself all over again, paying attention to nice little details, creating new temptations. In fact you should mix the two aspects, for too much pain or pleasure will not prove seductive. You are not repeating the first seduction, for the target has already surrendered. You are simply supplying little jolts, little wake-up calls that show you have not stopped trying and they cannot take you for granted. The little jolt will stir up the old poison, stoke the embers, bring you temporarily back to the beginning, when your involvement had a most pleasant freshness and tension. Never rely on your physical charms; even beauty loses its appeal with repeated exposure. Only strategy and effort will fight off inertia.

Age cannot wither her, nor custom stale \ Her infinite variety: other women cloy \ The appetites they feed; but she makes hungry \ Where most she satisfies.

—WILLIAM SHAKESPEARE, *ANTONY AND CLEOPATRA*

Maintain mystery. Familiarity is the death of seduction. If the target knows everything about you, the relationship gains a level of comfort but loses the elements of fantasy and anxiety. Without anxiety and a touch of fear, the erotic tension is dissolved. Remember: reality is not seductive. Keep some dark corners in your character, flout expectations, use absences to fragment the clinging, possessive pull that allows familiarity to creep in.

> *Men despise women who love too much and unwisely.*
> —LUCIAN, DIALOGUES OF THE COURTESANS, TRANSLATED BY A.L.H.

Sensing that the spell is broken, some targets may turn to another man or woman whose unfamiliarity seems exciting and poetic. Do not play into their hands by complaining or becoming self-pitying. That would only further their natural disenchantment once the seduction is over. Instead, make them see that you are not the person they thought you were. Make it a delightful game to play new roles, to surprise them, to be an endless source of entertainment. Play up the parts of your character they find delightful, but never let them feel they know you too well.

Maintain lightness. Seduction is a game, not a matter of life and death. There will be a tendency in the "post" phase to take things more seriously and personally, and to whine about behavior that does not please you. Fight this as much as possible, for it will create exactly the effect you do not want. You cannot control the other person by nagging and complaining; it will make them defensive, exacerbating the problem. You will have more control if you maintain the proper spirit. Your playfulness, the little ruses you employ to please and delight them, your indulgence of their faults, will make your victims compliant and easy to handle. Never try to change your victims; instead, induce them to follow your lead.

Avoid the slow burnout. Often, one person becomes disenchanted but lacks the courage to make the break. Instead, he or she withdraws inside. As an absence, this psychological step back may inadvertently reignite the other person's desire, and a frustrating cycle begins of pursuit and retreat. Everything unravels, slowly. Once you feel disenchanted and know it is over, end it quickly, without apology. That would only insult the other person. A quick separation is often easier to get over—it is as if you had a problem being faithful, as opposed to your feeling that the seduced was no longer being desirable. Once you are truly disenchanted, there is no going back, so don't hang on out of false pity.

Not only does the long, lingering death of a relationship cause your partner needless pain, it will have long-term consequences for you as well, making you more skittish in the future, and weighing you down with guilt. Never feel guilty, even if you were both the seducer and the one who now feels disenchanted. It is not your fault. Nothing can last forever. You have created pleasure for your victims, stirring them out of their rut. If you make a clean quick break, in the long run they will appreciate it. The more you apologize, the more you insult their pride, stirring up negative feelings that will reverberate for years. Spare them the disingenuous explanations that only complicate matters. The victim should be sacrificed, not tortured.

If a break with the victim is too messy or difficult (or you lack the nerve), then do the next best thing: deliberately break the spell that ties him or her to you. Aloofness or anger will only stir the other person's insecurity, producing a clinging horror. Instead, try suffocating them with love and attention: be clinging and possessive yourself, moon over the lover's every action and character trait, create the sense that this monotonous affection will go on forever. No more mystery, no more coquetry, no more retreats—just endless love. Few can endure such a threat. A few weeks of it and they will be gone.

Re-seduction

Once you have seduced a person there is almost always a lull, a slight letdown, which sometimes leads to a separation; it is surprisingly easy, though, to re-seduce the same target. The old feelings never go away, they lie dormant, and in a flash you can take your target by surprise.

It is a rare pleasure to be able to relive the past, and one's youth—to feel the old emotions. Add a dramatic flair to your re-seduction: revive the old images, the symbols, the expressions that will stir memory. Your targets will tend to forget the ugliness of the separation and will remember only the good things. You should make this second seduction bold and quick, giving your targets no time to reflect or wonder. Play on the contrast to their current lover, making his or her behavior seem timid and stodgy by comparison.

If you want to re-seduce someone, choose those who do not know you so well, whose memories of you are cleaner, who are less suspicious by nature, and who are dissatisfied with present circumstances. Also, you might want to let some time pass. Time will restore your luster and make your faults fade away. Never see a separation or sacrifice as final. With a little drama and planning, a victim can be retaken in no time.

Symbol:

Embers, the remains of the fire on the morning after. Left to themselves, the embers will slowly die out. Do not leave the fire to chance and to the elements. To put it out, douse it, suffocate it, give it nothing to feed on. To bring it back to life, fan it, stoke it, until it blazes anew. Only your constant attention and vigilance will keep it burning.

Selected Bibliography

Baudrillard, Jean. *Seduction*. Trans. Brian Singer. New York: St. Martin's Press, 1990.

Bourdon, David. *Warhol*. New York: Harry N. Abrams, Inc., 1989.

Capellanus, Andreas. *Andreas Capellanus on Love*. Trans. P. G. Walsh. London: Gerald Duckworth & Co. Ltd., 1982.

Casanova, Jacques. *The Memoirs of Jacques Casanova, in eight volumes*. Trans. Arthur Machen. Edinburgh: Limited Editions Club, 1940.

Chalon, Jean. *Portrait of a Seductress: The World of Natalie Barney*. Trans. Carol Barko. New York: Crown Publishers, Inc., 1979.

Cole, Hubert. *First Gentleman of the Bedchamber: The Life of Louis-François Armand, Maréchal Duc de Richelieu*. New York: Viking, 1965.

de Troyes, Chrétien. *Arthurian Romances*. Trans. William W. Kibler. London: Penguin Books, 1991.

Feher, Michel, ed. *The Libertine Reader: Eroticism and Enlightenment in Eighteenth-Century France*. New York: Zone Books, 1997.

Flynn, Errol. *My Wicked, Wicked Ways*. New York: G. P. Putnam's Sons, 1959.

Freud, Sigmund. *Psychological Writings and Letters*. Ed. Sander L. Gilman. New York: The Continuum Publishing Company, 1995.

———. *Sexuality and the Psychology of Love*. Ed. Philip Rieff. New York: Touchstone, 1963.

Fülöp-Miller, René. *Rasputin: The Holy Devil*. New York: Viking, 1962.

George, Don. *Sweet Man: The Real Duke Ellington*. New York: G. P. Putnam's Sons, 1981.

Gleichen-Russwurm, Alexander von. *The World's Lure: Fair Women, Their Loves, Their Power, Their Fates*. Trans. Hannah Waller. New York: Alfred A. Knopf, 1927.

Hahn, Emily. *Lorenzo: D. H. Lawrence and the Women Who Loved Him*. Philadelphia: J. B. Lippincott Company, 1975.

Hellmann, John. *The Kennedy Obsession: The American Myth of JFK.*
   New York: Columbia University Press, 1997.
Kaus, Gina. *Catherine: The Portrait of an Empress.* Trans. June Head.
   New York: Viking, 1935.
Kierkegaard, Søren. *The Seducer's Diary,* in *Either/Or, Part 1.* Trans.
   Howard V. Hong & Edna H. Hong. Princeton, NJ: Princeton
   University Press, 1987.
Lao, Meri. *Sirens: Symbols of Seduction.* Trans. John Oliphant of
   Rossie. Rochester, VT: Park Street Press, 1998.
Lindholm, Charles. *Charisma.* Cambridge, MA: Basil Blackwell,
   Ltd., 1990.
Ludwig, Emil. *Napoleon.* Trans. Eden & Cedar Paul. Garden City,
   NY: Garden City Publishing Co., 1926.
Mandel, Oscar, ed. *The Theatre of Don Juan: A Collection of Plays
   and Views, 1630–1963.* Lincoln, NE: University of Nebraska
   Press, 1963.
Maurois, André. *Byron.* Trans. Hamish Miles. New York: D. Appleton & Company, 1930.
———. *Disraeli: A Picture of the Victorian Age.* Trans. Hamish Miles.
   New York: D. Appleton & Company, 1928.
Monroe, Marilyn. *My Story.* New York: Stein and Day, 1974.
Morin, Edgar. *The Stars.* Trans. Richard Howard. New York: Evergreen Profile Book, 1960.
Ortiz, Alicia Dujovne. *Eva Perón.* Trans. Shawn Fields. New York:
   St. Martin's Press, 1996.
Ovid. *The Erotic Poems.* Trans. Peter Green. London: Penguin
   Books, 1982.
———. *Metamorphoses.* Trans. Mary M. Innes. Baltimore, MD:
   Penguin Books, 1955.
Peters, H. F. *My Sister, My Spouse: A Biography of Lou Andreas-Salomé.* New York: W. W. Norton, 1962.
Plato. *The Symposium.* Trans. Walter Hamilton. London: Penguin
   Books, 1951.
Reik, Theodor. *Of Love and Lust: On the Psychoanalysis of Romantic
   and Sexual Emotions.* New York: Farrar, Strauss and Cudahy,
   1957.

Rose, Phyllis. *Jazz Cleopatra: Josephine Baker and Her Time*. New York: Vintage Books, 1991.

Sackville-West, Vita. *Saint Joan of Arc*. London: Michael Joseph Ltd., 1936.

Shikibu, Murasaki. *The Tale of Genji*. Trans. Edward G. Seidensticker. New York: Alfred A. Knopf, 1979.

Shu-Chiung. *Yang Kuei-Fei: The Most Famous Beauty of China*. Shanghai, China: Commercial Press, Ltd., 1923.

Smith, Sally Bedell. *Reflected Glory: The Life of Pamela Churchill Harriman*. New York: Touchstone, 1996.

Stendhal. *Love*. Trans. Gilbert and Suzanne Sale. London: Penguin Books, 1957.

Terrill, Ross. *Madame Mao: The White-Boned Demon*. New York: Touchstone, 1984.

Trouncer, Margaret. *Madame Récamier*. London: Macdonald & Co., 1949.

Wadler, Joyce. *Liaison*. New York: Bantam Books, 1993.

Weber, Max. *Essays in Sociology*. Ed. Hans Gerth & C. Wright Mills. New York: Oxford University Press, 1946.

Wertheimer, Oskar von. *Cleopatra: A Royal Voluptuary*. Trans. Huntley Patterson. Philadelphia: J. B. Lippincott Company, 1931.